PSYCHIATRY
IN
BROAD PERSPECTIVE

ROY R. GRINKER, Sr.

*Chairman, Department of Psychiatry and Director, Institute for Psychosomatic &
Psychiatric Research & Training, Michael Reese Medical Center*

*Professor of Psychiatry
Pritzker Medical School
University of Chicago*

BEHAVIORAL PUBLICATIONS, INC.
New York

Library of Congress Catalog Number 74-13012
ISBN: 0-87705-231-x
Copyright © 1975 by Behavioral Publications, Inc.

BEHAVIORAL PUBLICATIONS, INC.
72 Fifth Avenue
New York, New York 10011

Printed in the United States of America
56789   987654321

Library of Congress Cataloging in Publication Data

Grinker, Roy Richard, Sr. 1900–
    Psychiatry in broad perspective.

    1. Psychiatric research. I. Title.
[DNLM: 1. Psychiatry. 2. Psychology, Clinical.
WM100 G867p]
RC337.G74   616.8'9'0072   74-13012

This book is not dedicated to a person or persons, but to an institution—The Michael Reese Medical Center—with which I have had a "love affair" for most of my academic life. Through successive administrations I have been given the maximum of freedom and opportunities, and the best of facilities and resources with which to carry on my work. All this plus a loyal staff and superb co-workers have made my career possible, and never did I entertain any invitations to move elsewhere. I hope that in some measure my productivity has justified the confidence placed in me.

CONTENTS

Preface   7
  I. From Magic through Religion to Science
     and Back Again   9
  II. The Development of Psychiatry
     from Philosophy and Psychology   23
  III. Theory in Psychiatry   33
  IV. The Researcher   61
  V. The Object of Inquiry in Psychiatry   69
  VI. Research Designing   81
  VII. Normality   101
  VIII. Biological Research   109
  IX. Early Experiences, Psychoanalysis
     and Intrapsychic Processes   119
  X. Social and Cultural Techniques
     Applied to Psychiatry   131
  XI. Stress: Adaptation, Defenses, Coping
     and Disease   143
  XII. Clinical Research   161
  XIII. Developing an Integrated Theory:
     The Example of Schizophrenia   175

XIV. The Role of Psychiatry in Society   217

XV. The Future of Research Psychiatrists
and Psychiatry   233

Index   247

PREFACE

In 1970 my birthday was celebrated at a banquet, following which a lectureship was established in my honor at the Michael Reese Medical Center. In addition, a book entitled *Modern Psychiatry and Clinical Research,* and edited by Daniel Offer and Daniel X. Freeman, was published by my good friend Arthur Rosenthal—then of Basic Books. It contained papers contributed by scientific friends and former students.

Two contributions among the splendid scientific papers continually reverberated in my mind. The first was Judith Offer's retrospective review of some of my investigations. These demonstrated the changing principles and methods of psychiatric research, all increasingly oriented toward systems or unitary theory and, unplanned but not emphasized, partial contributions to the problems of the schizophrenias on which I am now concentrating.

The second and most important impact was the final chapter of the collection, a paper by Judith Offer, Daniel Freedman, and Daniel Offer entitled "The Psychiatrist as Researcher." In my opinion, this chapter is an excellent, although brief, exposition of problems of psychiatric research.

In searching for a way to summarize my own 40 years devoted to research, I discarded the idea of reviewing the passing scene through episodes of my life. Rather, I decided to amplify the model of the Offer, Freedman, and Offer chapter by delineating the principles behind psychiatric research. Despite the many difficulties in exposition of a field that is a conglomeration of many sciences, I chose this method as more appropriate to the subject, although it required reading hundreds of articles and books from many disciplines (not all of which are included in the chapter references). In this examination I present the work of many other investigators, from whom I quote liberally along with a liberal selection from my own work. Attempts will then be made to synthesize principles, concepts and theories, working as closely to empirical data as possible.

This book will not be philosophical, not a cookbook of detailed methods and not a critical evaluation of individual contributions. Furthermore, it will not include much about principles of research applicable to the many psychiatric therapies, because of difficulties in controlling the many unknowable variables and the absence of hard data from few evaluations of results. Instead, it will focus on problems in clinical psychiatry, the center of systematic psychiatric research; in fact, clinical psychiatry is the organizer of psychiatric research, to which many disciplines from biogenics to sociology are vigorously contributing. It is my optimistic hope that current and future investigators will be stimulated and will profit from this exposition.

Roy R. Grinker, Sr.

I

From Magic through Religion to Science and Back Again

It may seem strange that a book concerned with the principles of research in psychiatry should be introduced by a discussion of magic and religion insofar as they relate to science. My logic rests on the fact that the triad of magic, religion and science represents phases in the evolution of ways of thinking about human mentation. Just as in ontological stages of development nothing is lost, each stage participating in the patterns of the higher levels, so magical and religious ways of thinking persist in science, particularly in psychiatry.

Furthermore, when an organism has attained a high level, and if that level is weakened, repudiated and to some extent abandoned, the lower levels may appear again, often with their original strengths. This phenomenon is quite similar to biological *dedifferentiation* under stress, with Jacksonian *devolution* when disease destroys the controlling highest nervous centers, and with Freudian *regression*.

We currently exist in an era when science is being repudiated because it has not improved the quality of life, except in terms of more conveniences and material benefits. Indeed, scientific discoveries have been used by industry and the military for products that are even destructive to life I do not subscribe to the notion of a generalized anti-intellectualism, but I observe an escape from some more evolved hierarchies of value systems to those of an earlier era. Mysticism, irrationality and drug-induced psychoses in the name of mind expansion, as well as "freaky" religious behaviors, are indications of regressions of levels of thinking. In addition, religious teaching, spiritual forms and psychophysical disciplines from the Orient are intriguing Western man, who is disenchanted by his traditional churches. This revolt against reason directly implicates the field of psychiatry, which attempts to replace irrationality by rationality.

When, where and how a jump step from other primates to man occurred is not known. It was associated with the development of a prehensile hand, an upright posture and verbal speech. Man's brain functions enabled him to become self-conscious and cognizant of his ontological past, his present and future. He moved from constant alertness and retreat based on fear, to attempts at active mastery of nature.

He first attempted to manipulate nature according to his own ideas through magic, as is so well described by Sir James Frazer.[1] Widely separated societal groups seem to have shared similar rituals, incantations and behaviors, even though names and details might have varied. This universality of magic is so striking that we can consider it a developmental stage of the species, rather than a characteristic based on personal or group experiences (Frazer, p. 304).

We still see manifestions of magical thinking in obsessive-compulsive personalities, in occupational rituals, in rules for initiation into some social groups and in many other situations. In most sciences, especially the behavioral sciences, we can observe how powerful magic is by the obsessive concentration on ways to neutralize it, e.g., strict adherence to paradigmatic designs and the endless preoccupation with counteracting bias by the use of tests for reliability.

Magic failed, so man began to rely on powerful, invisible human-like beings called gods, who lived on mountain tops. Each god had its own functional domain. They could be supplicated, and sacrifices were performed for them. These gods were portrayed as if they had human forms when living on earth, and love, procreation, anger and murder occurred in their familial transactions on high. Man, in creating gods, seems to have directly projected all human strengths and frailties and many other qualities onto separate, invisible divinities.

The next phase of human thinking involved the integration of all gods into One who represented the regulation and control of all part-qualities of human nature such as love, hate, envy, etc. through the leverage of love and punishment. God then became a strong father figure whose commandments were explicit, and who gave hope for security here and now, and in the hereafter. This monotheistic supraordinate regulation and control thus represented the functional integration of all the projections that had heretofore been laid onto individual deities. A single supernatural spirit had economic advantages in that one powerful father was enough, even though some subsequent religions returned to a family of gods.

The evolution of thinking into a religious faith did not necessarily involve complete confidence in a supernatural being who safeguarded man's security. Too often innocent people in tragedy cried out "why," but received no answer, so that the conflicts, frustrations and miseries of the twentieth century finally weakened formal religion associated with obedience and prayer. Today, for many people, "religion" has taken on a different meaning. One dictionary definition of the word includes, "The quest for the values of the ideal life, involving three phases: the ideal, the practice for attaining the values of the ideal and the theology or world view relating the quest to the environing universe."

The third phase of thinking we call science, a way of thinking that involves observations of the regularities of nature and their descriptions. Obstructions, persecutions and negative reactions to the scientific approach have dominated the history of man from Galileo to the present. But science is not free of religion as defined above. It is constantly involved in *faith* that the ultimate truth will be uncovered—so magical ideas and expectations persist in scientific biases. Religious faith is invested in science and its results, and in its hope of improving the human situation. Attempts at complete objectivity are never successful, and statements frequently made by scientists that they are "playing" with this or that implies their concern over failure.

The value systems of science, although directly related to the "ideal," have failed either directly or indirectly partly because scientific achievements have been misused for destructive purposes and because the good material life has not substituted for the values of the "golden era" of man.

We have clearly recognized that these disappointments have resulted in an anti-scientific attitude and a return to mysticism and magic. More important is the concept that "humanism" is separate from and in conflict with science. I shall later discuss this in detail as it applies to psychiatry, which also seems to be disintegrating into magic and religion in therapy and research, although the regression is designated by other names.

Gregory Bateson[2] has discussed the evolution of mind, in his *Steps to an Ecology of Mind,* from a somewhat different vantage point. By *ecology* he means the way ideas interact with one another, and *steps* are benchmarks or points of reference. He favors a process of deduction from the fundamentals or philosophy of science, rather than induction from data to hypotheses. Data, he correctly states, are not "raw," but are altered by recording and selection, and can only lead to heuristic explanatory concepts. He considers that the ultimate goal of science cannot be achieved by induction because form or pattern, not substance, depends on cybernetic or systems theory. We lack concepts and language to form a bridge across data, explanatory and fundamental concepts.

Objectivity as the ultimate goal of science is a misconception since our world is viewed subjectively through our sense organs or their extensions. Heisenberg's uncertainty principle was a blow to scientific omniscience, forcing us as observers always to define our position in time and space and to draw only probability conclusions.

Alexander[3] states that contemporary art uses magic and symbolism as a revolt against reason. Dostoevski put his revolt in the form of loss of freedom or becoming mad for the purpose of finding oneself. To prevent the collapse of Western civilization, Alexander *wishes* that the road of thinking would lead back to reality and reason; that the magical unconscious would yield to ego realism. Man has to accept the dread of individual existence, develop an internal sense of identity and a capacity to endure changes in values.

Huxley[4] considers that religion is a psychosocial imperative for man, concerned as it is with the problems of destiny, and involving the values of right and wrong. It satisfies the higher manifestions of human nature and values: art, love and intellectual comprehension. The fuller realization of all these life's possibilities are a sacred trust (p. 238).

Harley Shands[5] equates scientific materialism with experimentation (thesis), and mysticism (antithesis) with contemplation and meditation. In dialectic thinking these are not opposites, but continuous. The human condition is symbolic and the liberation from it and the verbal is mystical experience. In other words, transcendental reality is beyond words. Shands states that the scientific model excludes human feelings in its quest for objectivity, but form, the nature of reality, is experienced in feeling. The truly human is outside science, but within the transcendental state in continuity with the divine presence. There are patterns of knowing and behavior, meaning movement between internal schemas and outside objects, so that often words and objects come to mean each other and the subjective and the objective flow together in symbolic patterning, avoiding the tyranny of lineal concepts.

Shands holds that sentences are analogous to genes, words analogous to amino acids and letters analogous to chemical elements. Does the supraphysiological emerge from physiological mechanisms? Finally Shands states that protracted submission to discipline facilitates the return to the undifferentiated state of infancy where it all begins—a return to the beginning. It is not worth losing one's life over the statistically significant, says Shands.

Frazer pictures the web of thought as composed of threads of different colors: 1) black magic; 2) red religion; and 3) white science. The composition of the web changes over time, and today we are seeing more black, but no one can foretell the future color of the cloth. Looking at the present scene, Frank,[6] for example, states that all psychotherapy includes the common features of magic, religious conversion and thought reform. Another psychiatrist states that mysticism joins and unites, but reason divides and separates. Fromm[7] believes that millions religiously await the return of another promised utopia.

Those who do not return to religion, but who search for concepts beyond science, are more erudite in their approaches. For example, Frazer in "Spirits of the Corn and of the Wild," *The Golden Bough* series, states: "Abstract generalizations of science can never adequately comprehend all the particulars of concrete reality. The facts of nature will always burst the narrow bounds of human theories."

Carl B. Rogers[8] believes that thoughts and feelings are intertwined, and that beyond the impression of our senses there may be a deeper understanding and a larger field of knowledge unrelated to science. Science is only one pathway toward knowledge. Other pathways, according to Rogers, are Psi-phenomena, paranormal states and mysticism.

Other distinguished authors do not repudiate science in favor of magic and religion under the modern title of humanism, but attempt to reconcile them. Thus Teilhard de Chardin (quoted by Birx),[9] wrote: "I submit that the tension between science and faith should be resolved not in terms of elimination or duality, but in terms of a synthesis."

Millikan,[10] in his Terry lectures of 1927 discussed four phases of human psychic evolution: first, the 1) magical personification of nature, developing into 2) a God or spirit involved in love and the golden rule; next, 3) the God of law, order and harmony based on observation and experimentation on the orderliness of the universe (in this phase the individual is subordinated for the good of the whole); and 4) the conception of a world beyond the field of science. This encompasses hopes, aspirations, reflection of the meaning of existence and responsibilities. "Science contributes to religion if it is humble and not dogmatic."

Simpson,[11] in the Terry lectures of 1949, stated that evolution and true religion are compatible. "It is clear that science alone does not reach all truths, plumb all mysteries or exhaust all values and that the place and need for true religions are still very much with us." Man is more than nothing but an animal. He is part of nature with more intelligence, flexibility, individualization and socialization than any other animal, and is more adaptable and independent of his environment. His social organization is the basis of a new evolution. He searches for an ethic good enough to survive in harmonious adjustment with his fellow man and his environment. His search for knowledge and truth is his real religion (p. 5).

Harley Shands[5] states:

> Man, condemned to conscious awareness and the incessant and hopeless pursuit of certainty and security by the overgrowth of his data processing potentialities, is doomed to contradictory movement throughout, not only the life of the individual, but the life of the group and the life of the species. In one direction he seeks always new means of mastering, of understanding an objective world which is constantly expanded and constantly expanding as we learn more. But in the other direction, man is constantly seeking to drop the incessant struggle, to find—or find again —that blissful state in which ignorance prevents us from perceiving difference.
>
> Even in this latter struggle, however, we find the inevitable duality of method. The human being automatically, without trying, and to a radical extent, does re-discover or re-encounter states of communion in dreaming, but at the talion price: the bliss thus found is again ignorance, doomed to be lost in the moment of awakening as we resume the burden of conscious resistance and conscious objecting and objectifying. In the other direction, the human being seeks communion through often life-long intense discipline, with an incessant attempt to grasp the obviously impossible, to understand the obviously incomprehensible. Delivery from this discipline occurs in brief moments of ecstatic communion—characteristically, as we have noted above, in feelings reported as maximally intense visual experiences ("illumination"), but vision again paradoxically without seeing anything.

So we come to ethics and values. Clyde Kluckhohn and Henry Murray[12] define a "value-orientation" as a generalized and organized conception—which influences behavior

—of nature, of man's place in it, of man's relation to man, and of the desirable and nondesirable as they relate to man-environment and interhuman relations.

Florence Kluckhohn[13] outlines 5 questions pertaining to value orientations (pp. 83-93):

1. What are the innate predispositions of man? In other words, what is the definition that a people will give of basic human nature?
2. What is the relation of man to nature? (e.g., subjugation to, harmony with, or mastery over)
3. What is the significant time dimension? (e.g., past, present or future)
4. What modality of activity is to be most valued? (e.g., being, becoming or doing)
5. What is the dominant modality of men's relations to other men? (e.g., lineal, collateral or individualistic)

From the psychoanalytic point of view, Kohut has, defined, in various personal communications those psychological structures guiding toward higher goals against reluctance. The highest ideal is not passionate truth-finding, but a shift toward the expansion of self, helping to create empathy toward others.

On the other hand, Frankel states:[14]

I speak of irrationalism as a studied and articulated attitude, proudly affirmed and elaborately defended, which pronounces science—and not only science, but, more broadly, logical analysis, controlled observation, the norms and civilities of disciplined argument, and the ideal of objectivity—to be systematically misleading as to the nature of the universe and the conditions necessary for human fulfillment. Despite the new language, half jargon and half slang, in which this irrationalism is expressed, the actual assertions on which it rests can be found in classic treatises on mysticism and in the utterances of many traditional philosophers and poets. The breathtaking departures from the thought-ways of industrial civilization, or of Western civilization, that are announced each month or each week are simply updated and usually bowlderized versions of views that go back to the Greek mystery cults and the pre-Socratic philosophers Heraclitus and Parmenides.

The irrationalist's theory of human nature is steeped in the tradition of the dualistic psychology it condemns. It talks about "reason" as though it were a department of human nature in conflict with "emotion." But "reason," considered as a psychological process, is not a special faculty, and it is not separate from the emotions; it is simply the process or reorganizing the emotions, of setting up a plan for satisfying them, a scheme of relative priorities constructed in relation to the resources and constraints of surrounding circumstance.

Such discussions have a long history in philosophic writings. Cantril et al.[15] state that scientific progress is faced with its enemies—personal attitudes, interests, preconceptions, etc.—which cannot be ignored but must be faced courageously. Karl Pearson,[16] on the one hand, thought that the scientific method can train the mind to an exact and impartial analysis of facts. Whitehead[17] to the contrary states:

Judgments of worth are no part of the texture of physical science, but they are part of the motive of its production. Mankind has raised the edifice of science, because it has judged it worth while. In other words, the motives involve innumerable judgments of value. Again, there has been conscious selection of the parts of the scientific fields to be cultivated, and this conscious selection involves judgments of value. These values may be aesthetic, or moral, or utilitarian;

namely, judgments as to the beauty of the structure, or as to the duty of exploring the truth, or as to utility in the satisfaction of physical wants. But whatever the motive, without judgments of value there would have been no science.

The practical consequences of the modern concepts that all observations are transactional—that is, that they involve a transaction between the thing observed and the observer —is that we must take into account the values, traits and states of the observer. For example, in our researches on the Borderline Syndrome,[18] our observers were at various levels of experience, age and optimism. Since it was impossible to denote all the observer variables, we wiped out their differences by utilizing all those who served the patient over the whole 24 hours and reported on the same behavioral incidents. If the number of observers interviewed (15 to 20) and the number of subjects is large enough, reliability can be reasonably assured.

Globus,[19] in a tightly reasoned article, suggests a complementarity between mysticism and science:

> Perhaps the antithesis is primarily methodologic, in that mystical knowledge assumes a perspective proximal to one transformation boundary, whereas scientific knowledge assumes an objective stance distal to all transformation boundaries. The present account of the identity thesis in relation to the world-knot suggests that these perspectives are complementary. Further, the notion of complementary psychoevent and psychoneural identity formulations provides a rapprochement between humanistically oriented dualist views and symmetric scientific nomistic accounts. Thus, the scientist can maintain the "spirit" of dualism while in no way compromising his materialistic account by adopting complementary perspectives in relation to the transformation boundary. (page 1134)

Psychiatrists, who are historians of a special kind dealing with the past of individuals, find themselves deeply involved in the current conflict, which is steadily increasing in intensity, between psychiatric science and the mystique of so-called humanism. If we are to discuss principles of clinical research, it should be obvious that our ways of thinking and our view of man in nature should be made explicit.

I have therefore attempted to outline an hierarchy of thinking showing how extensions of earlier forms are maintained, how they influence the evolutionary more advanced forms of thought and how the more primitive forms reappear when the control of reason is weakened. Yet I do not believe that science is characterized by reason alone; rather, it is shaped as well by mysticism, magic and religion in the broader sense of those terms.

Those who derogate the latter speak of this influence as irrationality; those who approve call it humanism. Students of mentation seem to be on the battleground on which this conflict is becoming increasingly violent, dividing an already loose federation of competing schools into opposing camps. I have adopted the systems view that includes both, not as antagonistic but as complementary. Before I approach this problem I shall briefly describe the historical development of psychiatry.

REFERENCES

1. Frazer, J. G. *The golden bough: a study in magic and religion.* (3rd ed.) New York: Macmillan, 1935.
2. Bateson, G. *Steps to an ecology of mind.* San Francisco: Chandler, 1972.
3. Alexander, F. *The western mind in transition.* New York: Random House, 1960.
4. Huxley, Sir J. Social and cultural evolution. In S. Tax (Ed.), *Evolution after Darwin.* Vol. 3. *Issues in Evolution.* Chicago: University of Chicago Press, 1960.

5. Shands, H. C. *The war with words.* The Hague–Paris: Mouton, 1971.
6. Frank, J. D. *Persuasion and healing: a comparative study of psychotherapy.* Baltimore: Johns Hopkins Press, 1973.
7. Fromm, E. *Escape from freedom.* New York: Avon Books, 1965.
8. Rogers, C. B. Some new challenges. *American Psychologist,* 1973, **28,** 379–388.
9. As cited by Birx, H. J. *Pierre Teilhard de Chardin's philosophy of evolution.* Buffalo: Caniseus College, 1972.
10. Millikan R. A. *Evolution in science and religion.* New Haven: Yale University Press, 1927.
11. Simpson, G. G. *The meaning of evolution.* New Haven: Yale University Press, 1949.
12. Kluckhohn, C., & Murray, H. *Personality in nature, society and culture.* New York: Knopf, 1948.
13. Kluckhohn, F. Value orientations. In R. R. Grinker, Sr. (Ed.), *Toward a unified theory of human behavior.* (2nd ed.) New York: Basic Books, 1967.
14. Frankel, C. The nature and sources of irrationalism. *Science,* 1973, **180,** 927–931.
15. Cantril, H., Ames, A. Jr., Hastorf, A. H., & Ittelson, W. H. Psychology and scientific research III. The transactional view in psychological research. *Science,* 1949, **110,** 517–522.
16. Pearson, K. *Grammar of science.* (3rd ed.) London: Block, 1911.
17. Whitehead, A. N. *The aims of education.* New York: Macmillan, 1929.
18. Grinker, R. R. Sr., Werble, B., & Drye, R. A. *The borderline syndrome.* New York: Basic Books, 1968.
19. Globus, G. G. Unexpected symmetries in the "world knot." *Science,* 1973, **180,** 1129–1134.

II

The Development of Psychiatry from Philosophy and Psychology

The ancient Greek philosophers were deeply concerned with discovering immutable truths based on their idealistic musings with colleagues and students in group introspections.[1] They were concerned with their physical wellbeing, their social security and their immortal place in the universe. Peters and Mace[2] indicate three phases of these ancient thought processes: presystematic, systematic but prescientific and scientific.

Within the presystematic phase, superstitions, dogma and occasional flashes of wisdom could be found. What fascinates us in the systematic phase is their consistent preoccupation with the relations between mind and body. Although magic had been abandoned, there remained considerable admixtures of religion expressed through concern with the soul and its specific properties such as sensation, motion, imagination, passion, volition, etc.

Even in ancient times, shift in the practical application of man's approach to the disordered mind occurred fairly rapidly. At first there was exorcism by the priestly and religious philosopher, which was succeeded by exorcism *with* the use of medication. Finally there appeared the physician-philosopher who recognized that mental disorder was not something apart from the body, and that extramundane forces were not part of causality.

There is a surprise on reading Hippocrates's[3] (460–357 B.C.) statement: "Art is long, life short, opportunity fleeting, environment dangerous, judgment difficult, nor is it sufficient that the physician should attend to his work, but it is necessary also that the patient and those around him should attend to his work, but it is necessary also that the patient and those around him should do theirs, and external conditions generally adjusted to the same end." Could anyone today find a more succinct and intelligent statement of field theory, transactions and community psychiatry?

Even classifications of mental disorders were made, for example, by Aretueus of Cappadox[4] in 90 A.D.: epilepsy, melancholia, mania, phrenitis, alcohol and drug delirium, senile dementia and secondary dementia. Kraepelin was not the first! Without itemizing the many brilliant ancient philosophies that used introspection, and that ultimately recognized that mind was located in the brain and that there were levels of consciousness, let us just point out that all this came to an end with the death of Galen in 200 A.D. not to be revived until Vesalius in 1543.

Those most interested in the mind at first maintained a parasitic reliance on philosophy, but later gradually emancipated themselves by joining the natural sciences. At the same time philosophy became less an inquiry into the ultimate nature of reality, and more concerned with critical analyses of the concepts of science and of the common man. Philosophy clarified concepts, psychologists attempted to verify them.

Psychologists tended to separate themselves into schools between which great verbal battles raged. Helmholtz,

Wundt, Watson, James, Tolman, Hull, Freud and countless others, so well described by Roback,[5] each developed his own focus, theory and school. Today there are over 25,000 psychologists classified into many sections and publishing innumerable periodicals and books.

During the 14th and 15th centuries, physicians became more intensely interested in man's strivings, feelings and mental disturbances, but not until the Enlightenment of the 18th century did the spirit of humanism prevail sufficiently to liberate the psychotic from prison chains and a life of degradation.[6]

Physicians who cared for the "insane" at first served as custodians, but as nosological classifications were systematized they sought for "causes" within the brain.[7] For at least 45 years neuropathology claimed to be the "queen of the sciences" of psychiatry based on the equivalent to normal staining methods of Nissl and Alzheimer. When specificity of intracellular pathology was discredited, the organic approach shifted to neurophysiology and more recently to neurochemistry.

The modern era was introduced by the dynamism of Griesinger, Jackson, Sherrington, Pavlov, Charcot, Janet, Dejerine and finally by Adolf Meyer and Freud. Therapy shifted from custodial care to the rest cures of Weir Mitchell, to the use of drugs such as bromides and opium and then to moral therapy and psychotherapy. The cult of curability began in 1827, and has persisted in that each school of psychiatry claims its share of success in the battle against mental illness.

As early as 1852 Henry Holland[8] predicted the modern psychosomatic concepts:

> Human physiology comprises the reciprocal actions and relations of mental and bodily phenomena, as they make up the totality of life–scarcely can we have

a morbid affection of the body in which some feeling
or function of mind is not concurrently engaged—
directly or indirectly—as cause or as effect.

Although modern philosophers repeatedly evoke the
writing, and images of the ancient Greek philosophers in
attempts to reevaluate their meanings in the light of today's
problems, the living field has changed. The pragmatic approaches of the philosopher-psychologists such as James,
Pearce, Dewey, etc. indicated this shift.

After Descartes, who set up a dichotomy between the
reality of inner experience and impressions of the external
world of "reality," the subjective and objective became
separated, as did the concepts of idealism and empiricism.
When the positivists based their facts on sheer observation,
the oldtime philosophical interests waned and mathematics
increasingly came to symbolize conceptual and abstract entities, but not empirical data based on observations.

Psychology, after it veered away from philosophy and
joined the natural sciences, became increasingly concerned
with physiology, genetics and physical schema; in other
words, it became more reductionistic. As the ranks of psychologists burgeoned and split into various groups and
sections, most of them adopted the experimental method
with small, rigid, closed designs largely irrelevant to the
human situation. On the other hand, increasingly numbers
of psychologists became clinically oriented, as therapists
abandoning their scientific training to accept the medical
model.[9]

George Klein[10] has attempted to reconcile, in his personal credo, the ever-widening split between the so-called
scientific psychologists and those who choose to become
therapists:

I have drawn, I admit, a rather complex, perhaps even
bewildering sketch of a clinical psychologist—a fellow

who feels no need to call himself a clinical psychologist, yet is closely identified with the clinical attitude; who dislikes being called "a therapist" feeling his main calling is that of looking for lawfulness rather than curing people, yet who insists on doing psychotherapy; who prefers working in a clinical setting but at the same time considers the academic tradition of investigation and psychology's link to biological science pre-eminent in his professional identity; a fellow who believes too that what is good about clinical psychology, its orientation to the meaning of suffering should ideally be part of the working equipment of every psychologist; and that what is good about experimental psychology—its concern for controlled observation and for understanding the conditions of the occurrence of phenomena—should be part of the conscience of all psychologists.

Where all psychologists should join, he believes, is in the naturalist's love of phenomena including symbols, the highest level of human evolution.

When students of mental evolution discovered how great a role in science is played by symbols, they were not slow to exploit that valuable insight. The acquisition of so decisive a tool must certainly be regarded as one of the great landmarks in human progress, probably the starting point of all genuinely intellectual growth. Since symbol-using appears at a late stage, it is presumably a highly integrated form of simpler animal activities. It must spring from biological needs, and justify itself as a practical asset. Man's conquest of the world undoubtedly rests on the supreme development of his brain, which allows him to synthesize, delay, and modify his reactions by the interpolation of symbols in the gaps and confusions of direct experience, and by means of "verbal signs" to add the experiences of other people to his own [S. Langer, p. 22].[11]

Grinker[12] has outlined the phases of the symbolic system as follows:

1. The symbolic system which has resulted in the development of preconscious and conscious process as distinctly (?) human phenomena, developed by an evolutionary jump step from a system of signs.
2. There are ontological phases of learning, from body signs to visual imagery to primitive symbols to creative thinking, but the flow of information among these phases persists in all directions throughout life.
3. There are flexible transactional operations among these parts, so that all are involved in all forms of thinking.
4. All phases or parts of the symbolic system are in transactional relationship with outer reality and inner experience.
5. A disintegration of optimum or effective relations among parts of the symbolic system may lead to breaking off of transactions or connections and thereby lead to distorted thinking and behavior repression or sometimes to temporary acceleration of creativity.

Perhaps Margenau[13] sums up the current problems of epistemology when he points out that the scientist has tended to move away from reliance on solidly observable and inspectable phenomena, and toward abstract conceptualization. There is, however, a wide chasm between sense data and concepts that our minds create. Both signs and symbols seem to be fused into a union which we call reality. Observed facts are used as the basis of the superstructure of theories. He quotes Kant:

Concepts without factual content are empty. Sense data without concepts are blind. Therefore it is equally necessary to make our concepts sensuous, i.e. to add to them their object in intuition, as it is to make our intuitions, intelligible, i.e. to bring them under concepts. These two powers or faculties cannot exchange their functions. *The understanding cannot see. The senses cannot think.*

Thus, facts are blind until enlivened by ideas but ideas are empty until they receive factual confirmation.

Grinker[14] recently wrote:

> L. L. Whyte's[15] phrase "Unity in diversity and continuity in change" is exemplified by personality with considerable freedom of choice within social patterns of behavior to which it must at least partially conform. Yet both factors together constitute an open system or network with formative tendencies leading to change. Dualistic thinking, on the other hand, is static and oriented toward stability and permanence.
>
> Our objective sciences tend to isolate parts of systems and to observe, describe, and identify their functions as if they were set as parts of a machine. We gain a sense of security by "knowing" that what is will continue to be, even though our senses indicate that this is an illusion. Similarly, the background against which we view or focus on any part-function is considered to be steady even though it is constantly moving, albeit slowly. We try to keep our world in a steady state.
>
> Unitary thinking, on the other hand, considers that both parts and whole, both focus and background are constantly changing but are regulated by some form of organization that prevents dedifferentiation, focal cancerous overgrowth, internal psychological confusion, social chaos, or anarchy. Our problem is to identify the ways by which the organizational principle operates.
>
> There are cogent reasons why the scientific psychiatrist and psychologist and the social scientists should

lead the way toward unified thinking in their research, translating its philosophical abstractions into concrete operations. It is just because our particular system of study has become greatly extended to include many parts—from biogenetics to culture—and has exposed many interfaces with other systems—from education to world organizations—that we have the responsibility of leadership. This requires abandonment of ideologies, polarizations, and limited focusing on conflicts. Instead, we should develop an approach to systems and specifically concern ourselves with the properties and functions of organizational processes and their interfaces by employing unitary thinking, out of which our search for meaning may be furthered.

References

1. Alexander, E. G., & Selesnick, S. T. *The history of psychiatry.* New York: Harper & Row, 1966.
2. Kant, I. Cited by H. Margenau, in *Main currents in modern thought,* 1973, **127,** 163–171.
3. Hippocrates. Cited by J. R. Whitwell, *Historical notes on psychiatry.* London: H. K. Lewis & Co., 1936, p. 61.
4. Aretueus. Cited by J. R. Whitwell, *op. cit.,* p. 163.
5. Roback, A. A. *A history of American psychology.* New York: Crowell Collier, 1964.
6. Bromberg, W. *The mind of man: the story of man's conquest of mental illness.* New York: Harper & Row, 1937.
7. Deutsch, A. *The mentally ill in America.* (2nd ed.) New York: Columbia University Press, 1949.
8. Holland, H. *Mental physiology.* London: Longmans, Brown, Green & Longmans, 1852.
9. Grinker, R. R., Sr., Albee, G. W., Shacter, J., Garmezy, N., Thrasher, R. H., & Mensh, I. V. Emerging conceptions of mental health and models of treatment. *Professional Psychology,* 1971, **2,** 129–145.
10. Klein, G. S. Credo for a "clinical psychologist." *Bull. Menninger Clinic,* 1963, **27,** 61–73.

11. Langer, S. K. *Philosophy in a new key.* Cambridge, Mass.: Harvard University Press, 1942.
12. Grinker, R. R., Sr. Symbolism and general systems theory. In W. Gray, N. D. Duhl, & F. D. Rizzo, (Eds.) *General systems theory and psychiatry.* Boston: Little, Brown & Co., 1968.
13. Margenau, H. The method of science and the meaning of reality. *Main Currents in Modern Thought,* 1973, **29,** 163–171.
14. Grinker, R. R., Sr. The continuing search for meaning. *American Journal of Psychiatry,* 1970, **127,** 725–731.
15. Whyte, L. L. *The next development in man.* New York: Henry Holt, 1948.

III

Theory in Psychiatry

In the preceding chapter we have observed that psychiatry developed from philosophy and psychology, although from antiquity scholars concerned with mind-body relations and the nature of the soul were also interested in deviant behavior. Philosophers continually introspected and debated about theory, becoming segregated into multiple schools designated by the names of their founders. *The Encyclopedia of Philosophy*[1] contains eight volumes devoted to the schools and heroes of philosophy. These not only represent the evolution of scientific thinking, but contain nuggets that represent remarkable prescience of current theory.

Psychology, which split from philosophy, also developed great disputes and multiple schools of thought which defied a specific clear-cut image of human beings. Instead, according to Metzger,[2] "Psychology becomes a collection of correlations between all possible psychological facts including all physiological, physical, geographical, sociological, etc. facts which may be found in their vicinity." Metzger contends that psychology is no longer a young vital, progressive science, but seems to be in a state of crisis because it has entered the therapeutic field and is no longer exclusively engaged in science.

We may historically separate the concepts relating to psychotics from conceptualizations about patients with neurotic or psychosomatic disabilities. The two latter groups of people were recognized to be suffering from difficulties in coping with problems of living, and in the 19th century they were treated by support, direction and suggestion, with no attempts made to uncover inner causative agents. Drugs, such as opiates and bromides, were used copiously. Weir Mitchell,[3] after the American Civil War, placed his patients in "rest-cures" comprised of bedrest and high fat diets. The diets were based on the theory that fatigue had used up the fat in the myelin sheaths covering the nerve fibers.

Much earlier psychotic behaviors, on the other hand, were believed to represent possession by demons, and the female psychotic was frequently identified as a witch. Many were burned at the stake, others were incarcerated in jails and subjected to inhumane treatment until Pinel in France and Tuke in England liberated them.[4] But the asylum-hospitals that followed were little better. Visitors came to be amused by the characteristic atmosphere of "bedlam." Eventually, in the United States, a "moral" or humane treatment was instituted in the large state hospitals by psychiatrists.

This attitude began to weaken as the hospitals expanded to make room for the increasing number of patients, and only a few physicians became interested in psychiatry. Then many psychologists moved into the hospital. The main preoccupation of these physicians was classifying conditions into diagnostic categories whose labels were equated with prognosis. To jump ahead a bit, Kraepelin's[5] classification of the psychoses dominated psychiatry for years, and even now its remnants exist. But his was neither the first nor the last. Valuable at one time, Kraepelin's classification based on supposed outcome became a barrier to progress in psychiatry.

Psychiatry, continuing the tradition of its ancestors, philosophy and psychology, also began to fragment into schools based on therapeutic procedures resulting in specializations of methods (an attempt is made to define psychiatry later in this chapter). These eventually included individual, group, family and community therapy, pharmacotherapy, behavioral therapy, encounter groups causing more casualties than benefits, and existential therapy, along with suggestion, direction, support and reeducation. A dichotomy has developed in recent years between the so-called medical model practiced by psychiatrists, and the humanistic model fathered by psychologists such as Rogers[6] and Maslow.[7] In opposition to psychiatrists, they initiated great controversies and useless bitter debates (see chapter XIV).

Psychiatry as a medical specialty concerned with diagnosis, treatment and prevention has maintained therapeutic activity in behalf of the mentally and emotionally disturbed, but two ingredients necessary to a scientific discipline were missing. In the first place, there was and is no adequate theoretical umbrella under which to develop hypotheses. Secondly, there have been no good follow-up studies to evaluate the results of any form of therapy, so that we have no hard facts—although Strupp[8] and his colleagues have made several serious attempts. The number of moving and unexpected variables is so great that they are difficult to hold steady.

At least so-called moral treatment persisted, which in plain language means that the mentally ill were treated as human beings and not animals to be viewed through a cage for a fee. There was an attempt to separate the organic from the functional among the various syndromes; an attempt that now seems puerile, because all disturbances of function reside in an organic structure. Another error that still occurs is the attempt to separate exogenous or reactionary failures in coping, from endogenous or essentially biogenetic diseases. The fact that heavy biological loading requires only minor precipitating factors, and that mild genetic loading succumbs only to severe precipitating factors, is only now clearly recognized.

Each therapist usually applies to most patients coming his way the form of treatment for which he was trained by the school of his choice. But we are now aware that susceptibility, conflicts, coping and treatment methods are all dependent on differentiated specific aspects of the life cycle. Thus we have child, adolescent, young adult, middle adult and geriatric phases of the life cycle, each requiring special methods of diagnosis and treatment. There is more scientific validity to such classifications, than to treating each patient solely according to his *own* isolated problems (we shall discuss this later in more detail).

It is quite clear, according to the opinion of most laymen, that psychiatry as a medical specialty is entirely devoted to diagnosis and treatment. But psychiatry also belongs to the sciences—not to "our science," but to science in general. Science recognizes categories—not overlooking but minimizing the individual patient. The era of reports on "a patient with a case of—" is long since gone. Nor can it be said that research interferes with treatment. Clinical psychiatry as a science is a system of communications involving observations and descriptions of deviant behaviors and a collection of theories divisible into three component areas: biology, psychology and sociology, linked by an overarching general theory.

During the first twenty-five years of this century, the physical sciences occupied the attention of the reductionists in psychiatry. In the last thirty years, psychiatry has been dominated by psychoanalytic theory and methodology. In fact, young residents all wanted to be analysts, and therefore first-class citizens. As time went on, it became increasingly difficult to separate the wheat from the chaff in this discipline, since current analytic theory is a mixture of early Freudian ideas and his later modifications, with little deviation from Freud's statements on the part of his followers. Their repetitiveness, the lack of organization of psychoanalytic theory and the "movement" aspects, as well as the parochialism of psychoanalysis, weakened interest in the field. Nevertheless, despite the time, cost and energy devoted to psychoanalytic therapy and, in contrast, its meager therapeutic results, much of psychoanalytic theory is valuable and important and should be taught to the student. Then came a recrudescence of moral therapy—this time under its new label of milieu therapy—and the advent of community psychiatry, which has been overadvertised and overevaluated to the point where psychiatrists were expected to be social planners and social engineers.

Multidisciplinary research,[9] concerned with various phases of neurobiology including genetics and biochemistry, psychology of various types and anthropology, became popular. Stress research required a combination of these modalities, as did the temporary burgeoning and hopeful breakthrough of psychosomatic medicine. This required sophisticated statistics, to replace simple correlations, and the use of adequate programming for computer analysis. Psychiatry extended its boundaries beyond the comprehension of general psychiatry. Research, treatment and training in psychiatry became an extended field of multiple disciplines "riding madly in all directions."[10]

Psychiatry seems to abound in theories with varying distance from each other and from empirical data. Closer observation, however, reveals that most of these theories are attached to schools or sects. Often the assumptions are questionable, the theories vague and the hypotheses self-fulfilling. Systems of control and comparison are woefully lacking and follow-up studies are meager. Outcome theory based on course of treatment and results has yielded false information as, for example, in the descriptive term "dementia praecox" developed by Kraepelin. Abraham Kaplan[11] pleads for more theory, in order to raise questions that cannot be answered by assumptions. On the other hand, some investigators deny that they operate under the umbrella of any theory or that they use hypotheses in setting up their research designs. Such disorganized "fishing" efforts may, through serendipity, produce valuable results, but rarely and at great cost.

Theory is an organizer of existing knowledge for which certain assumptions are specified, stimulating the search for explanatory propositions that we call hypotheses. If the theory is internally consistent, alternative hypotheses may be entertained, all with empirical references and operational definitions. In brief, logical approaches to research require statements of assumptions based on past investigations or empirical experience, statements of theory, specified hypotheses and definitions of proposed operations. Yet, many researches are based on safe and popular concepts, expedient and practical objectives.

Theory and empirical research are closely intertwined. The former exists as an umbrella, receiving, giving and altering in reciprocal relations with the latter. Neither is productive without the other. This is true whether we begin deductively or inductively, for neither method of thinking can stand alone. Nor can we agree with reductionists who state that psychology is like a tapeworm whose tail is constantly being incorporated into physiology.

Paul Weiss[12] decries reductionism even when applied to a single cell, and he abhors words such as "regulators," "integrators" and "organizers." The component parts of the cell are interdependent and compensate for each other's failures. The behaviors of a cell cannot be accounted for except in terms of the cell's role as part of a system.

Reviewing the literature on research in psychiatry as a *field* is a difficult task. It would take a lifetime to become proficient in more than one or two of the disciplines that are necessary and ancillary to clinical psychiatry, although the general principles of each contributory science may be fairly well grasped. For example, psychology as a science is at least partially encompassed in seven thick volumes edited by Koch,[13] and for such areas as biogenetics, anthropology, sociology, etc., the massive amount of published material is scattered within many books and periodicals.

In the modern field-theories concerned with psychopathology, discussed by distinguished authors over the last thirty years, the same important concepts are endlessly repeated. Each author uses somewhat different words and provides a different emphasis, but the end result is the overriding notion of a field, a system, a unified theory sufficiently broad to encompass biopsychosocial man.[14/15/16/17]

Any overarching unified,[18] general systems[19] or field theory or metatheory which encompasses multiple levels of biopsychosocial processes requires multidisciplinary operations. Each discipline has its own divisions and subdivisions; its methods, directions and vocabularies that create barriers to communication.[20] But these barriers can be overcome. Wallerstein and Smelzer[21] give an example of the interpenetration of psychoanalysis and sociology. They stress the complementary articulation between disciplines to achieve a high rate of predictability and the avoidance of simplified assumptions and artificial boundaries with the "other" disciplines. They warn against idealization of each discipline and emphasize that different hierarchical levels have different functions and consequences. If problems are defined appropriately, costs and benefits understood, then value differences become apparent. In general, all disciplines use the language of behaviors; a language that we will discuss in greater detail in a later chapter.

Multidisciplinary groups tend to communicate in analogies in order to create models that, as Zubin[22] believes, have the power of pointing investigators to further research and then disappearing. "A model is a reconstruction of nature for the purpose of studying a given phenomenon. It is built by a process of abstraction, defining a parsimonious set of parameters that are intended to leave intact the essential aspects of reality, while removing distracting elements."[23] There is no end to the types of models possible, in addition to the traditional organic, hereditary-environmental, personality, developmental, social and cultural. What is sparse in all these, and probably many other, models is the lack of observational data and derived generalizations on which models of varying degrees of abstraction must be based.[24/25/26/27/28/29/30]

Zubin points out that these models of theories require study of the interactional processes among them. But Zubin correctly adds another approach to all others: the biometric model. I would warn that the "add on" does not mean at a later stage, but during the planning stage before research has begun.

There seems to be a reciprocal relationship between biochemical, pharmacological and psychological factors, for example in depressions. Starting at either arc of the cycle, any transaction may initiate the whole process. It can start with a biochemical alteration, or a psychological stress-stimulus, and the process can be the same no matter where it begins. The difficulty is in separating the psychological indices from the more basic elements of the process (up to the present we have felt that they must be studied as closely together in time as possible). The levels of complexity are great on both sides. Exact biochemical and rough clinical estimates are really not correlatable. Also, the biochemist has the responsibility for using the clinical phenomena as we now know them. It is true that in the future these may be modified, but at least what we have as our "information" now needs to be used.

The real problem is a systematic study of a system. The question is: are we all working on the same "what?" Do we know what we're working on? We have thought, as clinicians, that we have a responsibility for *defining* the "what" as well as we could. But the biochemist and physiologist also have a responsibility for *using* the "what" as we now can define it. If we do not do this, we cannot hope to answer the "how," the etiology, and the "why," the adaptive functions.

Dubos[31] decries the irrelevance of present day biology to the humanities when it concentrates only on physiochemical mechanisms. George Simpson,[32] the noted paleontologist, recounts the many characteristics common to all mankind and to other primates. At the molecular level, man hardly differs from the bacteria. By virtue of the development of language and the power of symbolization,[33] and his upright position, he has developed societies and cultures "unique in kind and complexity," which must be defined by the clinician.

Behaviorism in psychiatry has come to mean a special form of therapy, although Pavlov initiated the whole enterprise by scientific studies of conditioned reflexes in animals. In this country, behaviorists applied Pavlov's findings to humans in an attempt to understand their reactions to environmental stimuli without the interposition of consciousness; the head and its contents was simply a stuffed black box. Millon's[16] recent book contains a summary of the most important contributions to this field.

We, however, are only concerned here with the theories of behavior analysis which are based on empirical laws of learning. In essence, behaviors are characteristic of the parts and wholes of all living creatures. Man's socially adapted and pathological behaviors are learned, including his total bodily activities, his part-behaviors in facial expressions and gestures, his vegetative and endocrine activities and his verbal behavior.

Based on the assumption that physiological and psychological states are intimately linked, then one may learn to change one's physiological state through reinforced conditioning (so-called biofeedback techniques), with the result that psychosomatic illness may be unlearned. Here is a new area of research that needs more than anecdotal statements.

Behavior analysis is directed toward studying the observable data of human behavior, excluding unchangeable heredity and constitution or the internal psychological activities, but including environmental stimuli that change behaviors. According to Skinner, these are shaped by the effects of operant conditioning and positive reinforcement.[34] In a recent study of the Borderline we used behaviors as means of identifying types of "ego functions" without introspection or uncovering psychic phenomena. By selective reinforcement, some investigators have attempted to treat psychotics, autistic children and anxiety states. Others have used behavioral analysis as an alternative to current diagnostic classifications.

Janis[17] defines personality deviations which may be considered as the nodular focus of psychiatric research. Patterns of behavior and predispositions determine how a person will think, feel and act. Research is then oriented toward determining behavioral differences between personalities and changes within a person. This includes hypotheses tested empirically with methods of assessment, development, responses to stress and frustration, and types of conflicts and defenses against them.

Benjamin[35] states that prediction is a goal of science, a proposition with which most people would agree, but he also states that it is a major tool in personality-theoretical research. Thus, for Benjamin, prediction is a goal of theory and a method. He applies psychoanalytic concepts as a background, in fact the background seems to overshadow the prediction itself. Benjamin correctly states that the innate and the experiential interact in development and that the dichotomy "nature vs. nurture" is absurd. Maturation is an inherited biological process, but development is integrated with it to produce phenotypes. The sensory-motor behavior derived from maturation is the template on which the affects and defenses of infantile separation anxiety are based. The maturational rate determines how the separation anxiety will be experienced, since there are innate differences in drive organizations and ego functions. "The individual twists society's pattern of behavior to make his life style."

The maturational sequences, according to Gardner Murphy,[14] are organized in the total field of the environment as differentiation occurs, but old innate patterns adaptive at one time in evolution may be currently maladaptive. Koestler[36] indicates that all primates *learn* how to play, use tools, develop some kind of language, cooperate socially and learn to be aggressive.

Coelho and Rubinstein[37] write of social change and behavior indicating that the long human immaturity is used to *learn* adaptation to society and culture and, especially, adaptation to occupational models. Humans learn best in early years within emotionally rewarding emotional bonds —only later are visible social objectives important. These may, by changing too fast, upset the adaptive equilibrium. This is especially true in America where pluralism, pragmatism, veneration for change and a belief in the accretion of ideas (future orientation) is in contrast with European adherence to past tradition.

Jurgen Ruesch[38] indicates the differences between theory and model in that the former is abstract and can be coded in mathematical terms, the latter simulates events. There are many kinds of models, among which Ruesch chooses action. Information accommodates action for, as he states, "the proof of a scientific model rests with the testing of the proposed solutions in the field." Action models pertain to all kinds of human functioning, and their results usually indicate the need for change in the basic assumptions.

There are a few "peculiar" theories concerned with psychiatry or psychopathology. For example, the World Health Organization (W.H.O.) indicated that "Normality is a state of complete mental health and social well-being, not merely the absence of disease or infirmity." On the other hand, some psychiatrists[39] hold that there are no mental diseases, that society is totally to blame for man's problems in living. They emphasize the challenges of society rather than the essence of the failure of preparation to meet these problems.

We have indicated that the field or system involving man in nature has many internal and external parts. It would be helpful if we had an adequate classification of what kinds of disturbances occur in various situations, but our nosological classification is woefully lacking in accuracy.[40] This obstructs sorely needed epidemiological studies.

We have, however, indicated some of the parts of the system that correspond to various disciplines of inquiry. Anyone who has participated in multidisciplinary experiences is aware of the babble that ensues when theories are expressed in so many different vocabularies or jargons that it is taxing to each participant.[20] Furthermore, even when empirical—and therefore intelligible—data is presented by other participants, the resultant relief at such clarity is not necessarily accompanied by a capacity to evaluate the data's reliability or validity. In fact, such data are frequently overidealized. Recently the theories of the mind, of psychopathology, and personality, have been summarized by Millon[16] and Sher.[15]

How can we put them all together, when the field is so riddled with confusing language?—language that embodies some theoretical concepts of the system's control and regulation. For example, does the system operate out of the ego or superego of psychoanalysis;[41] or is it the universal principle of homeostasis;[42] or is it interpersonal behavior based on the personality or self-system; or is it the pleasure principle that organizes behavior, and fails in anhedonia? Rapaport[43] reviewing Lazlo's book, states that:

> If the systems view is to be a genuine input to science, the analytic method must be *extended* to encompass holistic characteristics of system rather than replaced by a set of ready-made, intuitively suggested concepts, which for all their heuristic appeal may be of questionable value as building blocks of rigorous scientific theory.

In the early 20th century, a small group of naturalists, including Child[44] and Herrick,[45] working on experimental animals developed a series of propositions on which much of our current process concepts are based. Briefly, they stated that whole living organisms mature by differentiation of primary undifferentiated structure-functions; living boundary structures are semipermeable and permit control of input and output; substructures of whole organisms exist in gradients under *central control or regulation.* Jackson's *final common pathways*[46] carry many processes, forming divergent internal sources to achieve near-identical actions; living organisms maintain homeostasis within a healthy range under conditions of moderate stress.

These and other paradigms derived from the biological sciences produced information detached from human problems. How do laboratory and behavioral researches dovetail, and how do regulations at various levels of organization interdigitate? These two questions within the general climate of appraisal of relevance led Bertalanffy to the quest for theories concerned with the unity of science, and especially of human behavior.[47]

Increasing attempts are now being made to develop unifying theories for all sciences, with the biological sciences in particular being related to other disciplines applicable to human behavior. It is as if systems analysis is searching for fitting empirical data and methods by which to test its concepts; and the extended and fragmented field of psychiatry is searching for appropriate general theory.*

Paul Weiss[48] expressed the idea:

> In breaking down the Universe into smaller systems, into the society, the group, the organism, the cells, the cellular parts, and so forth, we dissect the system: that is we sever relations, and then we try awkwardly and clumsily to restore those relations systematically but frequently very inadequately.

Again Paul Weiss:

> If we had come down from the universe gradually through the hierarchy of systems to the atoms, we would be much better off. Instead we now have to resynthesize the conceptual bonds between those parts which we have cut in the first place. (page 115)

A more elegant definition has been furnished by Boulding:[49]

> General systems theory is a name which has come into use to describe a level of theoretical model building which lies somewhere between the highly generalized constructions of pure mathematics and the specific

---

*Parts of the discussion that follows are abstracted from my unpublished "Ludwig von Bertalanffy Memorial Lecture" given in New York, November 1973.

theories of the specialized disciplines. The objectives of general systems theory can be set out with varying degrees of ambition and confidence. At a low level of ambition, but with a high degree of confidence, it aims to point out similarities in the theoretical constructions of different disciplines, where these exist, and to develop theoretical models having application to at least two different fields of study. At a higher level of ambition, but with perhaps a lower degree of confidence it hopes to develop something like a "spectrum" of theories—a system of systems which may perform the function of a "gestalt" in the theoretical construction. Such "gestalts" in special fields have been of great value in directing research towards the gaps which they reveal.

General systems theory is what may be called a metatheory; that is, a conceptual overarching global theory that embraces several limited theories. These are the parts of the total system. These theoretical parts may be grouped, according to John Spiegel,[50] into *constitutional*, which concerns the internal structure-function of the system; *integrative*, which functions to relate the parts to the whole and prevent their disintegration or fragmentation; and *determinants*, that describe the function of the system in relation to other external systems.

Systems do not develop *de novo* because they and their parts have a past that remains part of their present, even though partially obscured. A process of maturation and development characterizes both living and conceptual systems. An appreciation of the ontogenic system must include isolating not only the factors concerned with growth, but also the timing of critical periods. Within the system, phases of the individual lifecycle of health and illness from birth to death have their own structure, function, susceptibilities, coping mechanisms and predominate types of degradation.

Parts of the systems come into being by a process of *differentiation* from an undifferentiated whole. These parts may be described in various ways depending upon the position of the observer and the resolving power of the observer's instruments. We could include the confluence of cells into individual organs and organ systems, the communicating systems of hormones, enzymes and the nervous system, the psychological system or mentation which extends beyond structure-function and the social and cultural systems learned or incorporated within psychological functions. Obviously, many more and finer subdivisions or subsystems may be included.

Each differentiated part subserves special functions in relation to each other and to the whole by some form or regulation. In this sense, they function in cooperation, but they are also in conflict or antagonism. These vectors of synthesis and fragmentation usually function adequately through opposing systems of enzymes and antagonists, nervous facilitation and inhibition, negative and positive feedback and by quantitative and temporal gradients.

From a single subsystem, which strain may cause to disintegrate functionally, to all subsystems and eventually to a total response, stress responses progressively spread and increase. The result is a multiplicity of circular and corrective processes between subsystems which are oriented toward stabilizing the organism and maintaining its integration. An intensification of activity occurs when strain becomes too severe, and eventually the pattern of behavior partially resumes its primitive infantile total functions when the subsystems which have been fractionated or differentiated out of the whole are no longer able to handle the strain. At first, stress stimuli facilitate defenses, but when continued and increased they disrupt and ultimately cause dedifferentiation. When the differentiated systems are under critical strain, the whole takes over and earlier patterns return.

Whether the organism reacts as a primitive whole before differentiation, or has been reduced by excessive stress to a dedifferentiated whole, the somatic and psychic systems are in a constant state of transaction with each other. Concomitant somatic and psychological action patterns probably occur as the result either of lasting traumatic impressions made upon a total system before differentiation, or as the result of current stress forcing regression to that state.[51/52]

As parts of a system become differentiated, they do not separate as in primary fission. Instead they constitute parts of a system characterized by a totality of elements organized by some form of central *regulation* that maintains integration or, in other words, functions against dedifferentiation. In embryonic phases, such a regulator functions to integrate the differentiating parts in proper temporal sequence. Within the functioning organism, local feedback circuits maintain homeostatic balance. The cerebral cortex regulates somato-sensory activities in many ways, but essentially in starting and stopping action, relinquishing further control to lower levels. In psychological terms, ego functions maintain a balance among the pressures of needs, desires and coping behavior.

Sometimes subsystems break out of control and the whole system decays. In other cases, the regulator may be congenitally weak or crippled by drugs, disease or fatigue. An example of the latter is the syndrome of ego depletion[53] during war. The soldier's horrible experiences destroy or weaken the compromises he has made between biological drives and reality. As a result of a breakdown of such psychological regulation, the soldier regresses to apparently more immature coping attempts.

It is not implied that functions of subsystems, their regulation or whole system, are rigidly and exactly programmed. There is an extensive range of successful *homeostatic* functions, wider in the young, narrower in the old. Failure results from activity exceeding these ranges.

For regulation and control we have always needed the concept of a higher level of psychological control; the absence of which has been a deficit in psychoanalytic theory. This may be a "self-system," which has so clearly been demonstrated by psychohistorical studies. How could the aggressive, vicious components of Gandhi's lifelong psychopathology have been controlled to preach love and abstinence, unless he were possessed of a supraordinate control that developed far later in life than during childhood, adolescence or young adulthood. Other examples of such late-appearing control have been described in Luther's and Jefferson's lives as well. These self-systems grow and change during middle adult years through social and cultural experiences that often fit the man for the task at hand.

Hierarchies are dependent on higher levels maintaining a regulatory dampening control over lower levels; but as higher levels weaken they release from inhibition the functional independence of lower levels. This corresponds, as previously stated, to the Jacksonian concept of evolution and dissolution of functional levels of the nervous system.

Theories of *communication* depict energy exchange as the basic process. There is no doubt that in living somatic systems this is largely correct. When, however, we proceed to the psychological system, although its fuel is dependent on energy furnished by the soma, its processes are conducted by means of communication of information. Living systems have *boundaries* which, in contrast with nonliving systems, are semipermeable—permitting substances and information to proceed in either direction. Information may be described by a variety of vocabularies such as those of mathematics, logic, linguistics, etc.

Information in open systems corresponds to negative entropy, in that it organizes and consolidates the chaos of multiple stimuli into meaningful data. In other words, organisms do organize and counteract the degradation of life.

No longer is it possible to maintain the mechanical view of man as passively incorporating mass or simply reacting to stimuli.

As an active personality system, man seeks goals for more than the gratification of his biological needs. He also searches for new goals. But the linkages among subsystems and systems occur in informational processes. These have only become possible for the whole organism because man has created, uses and modifies *symbolic systems* that are the bases for his more complex and flexible adaptive and creative acts.

Symbolic systems are not linear, nor are linear explanations valid in cause and effect explanations. Instead, we use the concept of *transactional* communication in which reverberating, corrective, circular systems of behaviors at all levels are possible.

Systems have evolved and they are born, develop and decay. Their position in this cycle of events is not always easy to determine. Dynamically, as organistic complexity evolved, systems became subsystems of larger systems, environments became part of expanding systems from cell to cosmos. In contrast, as systems decay they break up so that their subsystems became free and separately functioning systems.

The function of a system should be viewed in relations to other whole systems, as, for example, the personality system in relation to society or culture, or one social system with another. Herein lies purpose or teleology: "Teleology is a lady without whom no biologist can live. Yet he is ashamed to show himself with her in public."[54]

Abstractions, concepts and theories are useful tools, not facts of "real nature." They organize experiences but do not describe their real essence. Experience with empirical phenomena are the real test of knowing. Since techniques vary with each system, operations cannot be described by generalizations.

Theories serve heuristic purposes and are never meant to endure should they be shown to be internally inconsistent and fruitless in generating testable hypotheses. A theory of systems should do more than furnish satisfaction for believers as if it were a religion. General systems theory has had its share of criticism on this score, especially because it has introduced a new language, applicable to its role as a metatheory, highly abstract and far removed from empirical data. One critic asks the question "So what?" "It only establishes analogies among levels of organization or a number of systems and contributes no real progress." Yet, analogies are indeed significant sources from which to create new approaches to problem areas; one only has to listen to multidisciplinary conferences to hear etiological "hunches." Symbolic thought is indeed analogical thinking for the most part, and one of its creations has been the analogue computer.[55]

General systems theory has no methodology, as do no other theories, but it does establish a paradigm or outline a way of thinking of relationships, of parts and wholes and of inputs and outputs. Furthermore, if adequately demonstrated by one of several models, it enables the observer or experimenter to identify his position among a vast number of variables. Although isomorphism has been accentuated as a characteristic of living systems, it in no way denies that individual processes, levels, hierarchies or subsystems have, in addition to common properties, specific functions and lawful regularities differing from each other.

Theories should not be confused with data or used as their substantiation, as we have experienced interminably in psychoanalytic publications in which the language of theory and data form a confusing mixture. Instead, theory orients the observer toward a search for empirical relevancies on which the theory depends for its continued existence.

Nevertheless, a valid criticism against general systems

theory is the premature mathematization indulged in by several theorists, turning away those who cannot understand such language. As yet it may be too abstract or, on the other hand, some may display confidence in formulae instead of searching for empirical data.

According to Bennett:[56]

> There are two ways of dealing with complex, or multivariate, problems. One is to introduce arbitrary simplifications so that we can use the techniques of analysis that may be available. This is the mathematical approach. The other is to accept the complexity as to an irreducible element in the situation and search for a structure or pattern that will enable us to examine it as a whole. This is the systematic approach.

Before considering the relevance of general systems theory to clinical psychiatry, we should again attempt to define psychiatry as clearly as possible in order to know its component parts and its extent, and to differentiate psychiatry as a medical clinical specialty from psychiatry as a science. This is especially true since the entire field is rapidly evolving, extending and developing interfaces with increasing numbers of other specialties and systems. Unfortunately, as Shepherd[57] states: "During the past fourteen years, I would maintain that the expanding role of the psychiatrist has far outstripped the gains in established knowledge."

But psychiatry is a specific science only insofar as it is concerned with a particular system of verbal, written, gestural and behavioral communications characterizing observer-subject (therapist-patient) transactions. It is in addition a conglomerate of many sciences involved in the study of human behavior, including biological, psychological and social sciences. Since man is a biopsychosocial creature, psychiatry must include these sciences as part of the total system characterized by whatever variables are in focus at the time. Likewise, the applications of these parts and the total system have become so extended that psychiatrists have been likened to pioneer riders searching for fences that bound their territories (Grinker).[10]

Gradually more and more psychiatrists became interested and organized their own special groups, hoping to communicate in a common language consonant and not disjunctive with their own biological, psychological and social models. They were tired of senseless controversy about who knows the cause, they became convinced of multicausality and reciprocal relations rather than linearity of cause and effect. As a result, the probabilities of a systems approach were enhanced. This is not to assume that any scientist could cover the entire field, but he could feel more comfortable knowing where he was, instead of endless riding around in search of boundaries.

It seems as if psychiatry—or really, psychiatrists—were divided into one group composed of therapists, including psychotherapists, somatotherapists or sociotherapists,[58] and another group involved in research conducted by scientific psychiatrists. This is not to assume that one works in the laboratory and the other in the clinic. Both are to some degree therapists and investigators. But so far as the public and the vast majority of physicians are concerned, psychiatry conforms to the medical definition of a specialty.

After World War II, the focus of concern transcended the individual, a process continuing with rapid acceleration as a product of the times. Disciplines began to form multidisciplinary research groups, which were not really woven together but operated, with great difficulty, within a relatively broad, or absent, unified framework.[9]

Sometime in the latter part of the 1950's research and clinical psychiatrists became self-conscious when they suddenly discovered that psychiatry was an integral part of the vast field of the behavioral sciences. Ideas of unified or systems theory seem to furnish answers in their concepts of openness, communications, transactions, homeostasis and isomorphism.[59]

In separating the practice of clinical psychiatry from psychiatry as a science, we are dealing with a weak dichotomy because clinical psychiatry can be approached scientifically and the sciences that form the system of scientific psychiatry are ultimately concerned with deviations in human behavior and require clinical contact and expertise in eliciting behavioral, cognitive and affective data. The data of the basic sciences and those at the psychological level supplement each other. Unfortunately, life histories of patients reveal considerable diversity, and general principles are difficult to abstract. In other words, it is difficult to separate what is individual and incidental from what is general and essential, thus making a system of classification extremely difficult (nomothetic and ideographic).

Caws[60] states:

> The most useful conception of the unity of science seems to me to lie somewhere in the middle of the triangle defined by the reductive, synthetic, and encyclopedic conceptions. Where reduction can be done usefully, it should be done; where isomorphisms can be found they should be found, and where disciplinary barriers to communication can be broken down, they should be broken down. What I have been chiefly criticizing here is apriori approach to this problem, the assumption that there must be isomorphisms, the assumption that every science must fit into some rational order of the sciences. What I should wish to substitute for this is an empirical approach—not the claim that isomorphisms are necessary, but the recognition that they are possible, and to resolve to search for them wherever they occur. If a direct bridge is thus built between physics and biology, or between crystal growth and population movement, it is not because

there *had to be* a bridge but because there *happens to be* one which somebody had the sense to exploit.

Where there is no bridge or at least bridging language, analogy is still possible and stimulating. For example, we may analogize social institutionalization with psychological internalization. Emerson[42] analogizes the gene with the symbols of culture and Parsons the human incest taboo with sex differentiation at the organic level.

Attempts can be made, however, to interdigitate general systems theory with some aspects or parts of psychoanalytic theory—though not all, especially since psychoanalysis is still a hodgepodge of unrelated concepts, old and new, good and bad, productive and handicapping. For example, topological theory identifies symbolic systems (unconscious, preconscious and conscious) in terms of their positions in relation to conscious awareness.

Are we able to utilize general systems theory in all our clinical investigations by extracting hypotheses subject to observational or experimental proof? The answer is "no." Rarely, if at all, are we able to use the total theory or to even envisage total wholeness. Although we are able to define some special structures and some temporal functions and avoid most hierarchies, we still must limit ourselves to parts of systems or, better said, to small systems. But we can, indeed, know where we are in perceived reality and recognize some steady states. In most investigations general systems theory has limited practicability, depending on the research focus.

To recapitulate, we should ask ourselves several general questions, a few of which are outlined. What is the nature of the deficit or of the regressive dedifferentiation? What parts of the total biopsychosocial system are most involved or most vulnerable? Is the deficiency some general organizational process? What are the appropriate stress-stimuli and their meaning for survival? What and when are the earliest indicators of differences? How do we separate the essential primary process from its secondary elaborations or adaptations? Is anxiety as a quality an inherent or experiential difference? Can response-specifity to ordinary challenges, artificially induced stress-stimuli or historical data be determined? These and many other questions become important in clinical research programs oriented toward studying "process" rather than "content," and are the basis of selection from the wide variety of individual projects focusing on parts of the total system.

REFERENCES

1. Edwards, P. *The encyclopedia of philosophy.* New York: Macmillan, 1967.
2. Metzger, W. Do schools of psychology still exist? Paper presented at the 36th Japanese psychological association annual meeting. Osaka, Japan: Osaka University, 1972.
3. Mitchell, S. W. *Fifteenth anniversary address.* Trans. Amer. Medico-Psychol. Assoc., 1894.
4. Alexander, F. G., & Selesnick, S. T. *The history of psychiatry.* New York: Harper & Row, 1966.
5. Kraepelin, E. *Clinical psychiatry.* (7th ed.) Translated by A. Ross Deifendorf. New York: Macmillan, 1921.
6. Rogers, C. *Client-centered therapy.* Boston: Houghton Mifflin, 1951.
7. Maslow, A. G. *Motivation and personality.* New York: Harper, 1954.
8. Strupp, H. H. Basic ingredients of psychotherapy. *Consulting and Clinical Psychology,* 1973, **41**, 1–8.
9. Luszki, M. N. *Interdisciplinary team research, methods and problems.* New York: New York University Press, 1958.
10. Grinker, R. R., Sr. Psychiatry rides madly in all directions. *Archives of General Psychiatry.* 1964, **10**, 228–237.
11. Kaplan, A. *The conduct of inquiry.* San Francisco: Chandler, 1964.

12. Weiss, P. The cell as unit. *Journal Theoretical Biology,* 1963, **5,** 389–397. And Weiss, P. *The science of life.* Mt. Kisco, N.Y.: Futura, 1973.

13. Koch, S. (Ed.) *Psychology: a study of a science.* Vol. 5. New York: McGraw-Hill, 1959.

14. Murphy, G. *A biosocial approach to origins and structures.* New York: Harper Bros., 1947.

15. Sher, J. (Ed.) *Theories of mind.* New York: Free Press of Glencoe, 1962.

16. Millon, T. (Ed.) *Theories of psychopathology and personality.* (2nd ed.) Philadelphia: W. B. Saunders, 1973.

17. Janis, I. L. *Personality: dynamics, development and assessment.* New York: Harcourt, Brace & World, 1969.

18. Grinker, R. R., Sr. *Toward a unified theory of human behavior.* (2nd ed.) New York: Basic Books, 1967.

19. Bertalanffy, L. M. General systems—a critical review. *General Systems* 1962, **7,** 1–19.

20. Kruse, H. D. (Ed.) *Integrating the approaches to mental disease.* New York: Hoeber-Harper, 1957.

21. Wallerstein, R., & Smelzer, N. Psychoanalysis and sociology. *International Journal of Psychoanalysis,* 1969, **50,** 693–716.

22. Zubin, J. On the powers of models. *Journal of Personality,* 1952, **20,** 430–439.

23. Zubin, J. Scientific models for psychopathology in the 1970's. *Seminars in Psychiatry,* 1972, **4,** 283–296.

24. Maslow, A. *Toward a psychology of being.* (Rev. ed.) New York: Van Nostrand, 1968.

25. Havens, L. L. *Approaches to the mind.* Boston: Little, Brown, 1953.

26. Kallmann, F. J. *Heredity, health and mental disorder.* New York: W. W. Norton, 1953.

27. Williams, R. J. *Biochemical individuality.* New York: John Wiley, 1956.

28. Sheldon, W. H. Constitutional psychiatry. In T. Millon (Ed.), *op. cit.*

29. Goldstein, D. *The organism: a holistic approach to biology.* New York: American Book Co., 1939.

30. Kety, S. S. Current biochemical approaches to schizophrenia. *New England Medical Journal,* 1967, **276,** 325–331.

31. Dubos, R. Humanistic biology. *American Scientist,* 1965, **53,** 4–19.
32. Simpson, G. S. The biological nature of man. *Science,* 1966, **152,** 472–478.
33. Royce, J. R. (Ed.) *Psychology and the symbol.* New York: Random House, 1965.
34. Evans, R. I. *B. F. Skinner: the man and his ideas.* New York: E. P. Dutton, 1968.
35. Benjamin, J. D. The innate and the experiential in child development. In H. W. Brosin (Ed.), *Lectures on experimental psychiatry* (Proceedings of the Pittsburgh Bicentennial Conference), Pittsburgh: Pittsburgh Press, 1961.
36. Koestler, A., & Smythies, J. R. (Ed.) *Beyond reductionism.* Boston: Beacon Press, 1969.
37. Coelho, G. V., & Rubinstein, E. A. *Social change and human behavior.* Washington, D.C.: National Institute for Mental Health, 1972.
38. Ruesch, J. Action models. In G. F. D. Heseltine (Ed.), *Psychiatric research in our changing world.* Amsterdam: Excerpta Medica Foundation, 1969, p. 126.
39. Szasz, T. *The myth of mental illness.* New York: Hoeber, 1961.
40. Hoch, P. H. *Diagnosis in clinical psychiatry.* New York: Science House, 1972.
41. Spitz, R. *A genetic field theory of ego formation.* New York: International Universities Press, 1959.
42. Emerson, A. Dynamic homeostasis: a unifying principle in organic, social, and ethical evolution. *Scientific Monthly,* 1954, **78;** 67–85.
43. Rapaport, D. Review of E. Laszlo, *The systems view of the world.* In *Contemporary Psychology,* 1973, **18,** 371.
44. Child, C. M. *Patterns and problems of development.* Chicago: University of Chicago Press, 1941.
45. Herrick, C. J. *George Ellet Coghill naturalist and philosopher.* Chicago: University of Chicago Press, 1949.
46. Jackson, H. Croonian lectures on evolution and dissolution of the nervous system. *British Medical Journal,* 1884.
47. Bertalanffy, L. M. General theory of systems: application of psychology. *Social Science Information,* 1967, **6;** 125–136.

48. Weiss, P. Discussion in R. R. Grinker, Sr. (Ed.), *Toward a unified theory of human behavior.* New York: Basic Books, 1956.
49. Boulding, K. General systems theory: the skeleton of science. *General Systems,* 1956, **1**; 11.
50. Spiegel, J. P. Transactional theory and social change. In D. Offer, J. L. Offer, & D. X. Freedman (Eds.), *Modern psychiatry and clinical research.* New York: Basic Books, 1972.
51. Grinker, R. R., Sr. *Psychosomatic research.* New York: W. W. Norton & Co., 1953. (Rev. ed., New York: Jason Aronson, 1973).
52. Grinker, R. R., Sr. *Toward a unified theory of human behavior.* (2nd ed.) New York: Basic Books, 1967.
53. Grinker, R. R., Sr., & Spiegel J. P. *Men under stress.* New York: Blakiston, 1945. (Reissued, New York: McGraw-Hill, 1963).
54. Brueke, C. Cited by W. Cannon, *The way of an investigator: a scientist's experience in medical research.* New York: W. W. Norton & Co., 1945.
55. Colby, K. M. Research in psychoanalytic information theory. *American Scientist,* 1961, **49**; 358–369.
56. Bennett, J. G. Total man: an essay in the systematics of human nature. *Systematics,* 1964, **1**; 282–310.
57. Shepherd M. A critical appraisal of contemporary psychiatry. *Contemporary Psychiatry,* 1971, **12**; 303–321.
58. Strauss, A., Schatzman, L., Bucher, R., Ehrlich, D., & Sabshin, M. *Psychiatric ideologies and institutions.* New York: Free Press of Glencoe, 1964.
59. Ruesch, J., & Bateson, G. *Communication: the social matrix of psychiatry.* New York: W. W. Norton & Co., 1968.
60. Caws, P. Science and system: on the unity and diversity of scientific theory. *General Systems,* 1968, **13**; 3–20.

IV

The Researcher

Observations and questionnaires derived from investigators in any scientific field reveal that they do not constitute a homogeneous group. A wide variety of personalities, attributes and motivations and range of talents are involved in research. Despite the efforts by Roe[1] and others, no common personality features have been recognized, although differences conducive to the choice of disciplines seem to be operative. For example, investigators in the exact sciences and the life sciences differ significantly in their psychological organization. Yet there are many explanations for what makes a researcher and what he chooses for his objectives.

Some psychoanalysts attribute the drive for knowing and learning more about their discipline to unsatisfied infantile oral needs and curiosity. Infants certainly repetitively examine strange objects with their fingers, gaze long and hard at new objects and finally put them in their mouths. All but the sick and damaged perform these acts. Later in childhood almost everything new and strange evokes the question "why." Each answer provokes a new "why" almost automatically and it seems as if the child is less interested in the answer than in maintaining communications.[2] Finally, the parent reaches his level of tolerance and closes the system.

There are some children whose curiosity about the external world demonstrates a more focused interest. Their questions include: "How does it work?" and "What is it for?" This suggests a primitive scientific attitude that should be nurtured to develop into a later mature form. The experience of many educators would indicate that such nurturance is more frequent in families including parents or relatives with a successful professional or academic background. Added incentive arises when the families's system of values included an altruistic concern for the future of mankind.

It seems as if most healthy children reach a stage of development when they ask to "do it myself," and do it, without fear of ridicule. Unless their parents obstruct their innate creativity, they are not frightened by the unknown and later attempt to resolve the dichotomies imposed by current social concepts. The creative youngster attempts to put things together, the precursor of integrative or unified thinking. This is the "fun" experienced by the future investigator.

There is not sufficient information to determine how significant the economic status of the nuclear family is, in relation to an offspring's choice to pursue nonmaterialistic goals. In our experience, this is not an important variable because many scientists stem from economically lower-class families, and a wealthy background frequently produces a noncreative, hedonic wastrel with poor motivation. In any case, current academic salaries do not demand sacrifices of a decent income and little sacrifice of materialistic comforts.

Interest in science is a commitment to change and may be linked to a modicum, but not destructive, adolescent rebellion against the existing establishment and authoritative ideas. Perhaps the innate logical structures of the mind expressed at various levels of maturity may lead to a type of precision or a special quality of perception that demands revision of our loose ordering of the nature of mind and matter.

Another psychological faculty includes the capacity for temporary regression in the service of the ego, which leads to a rich fantasy life for which temporary isolation from the buzzing noise-pollution of the crowd is required. Some creative scientists suffer attacks of depression and produce their best work as they are emerging from their depressive regression. In this phase they excel in the capacity to synthesize and generalize. I do not want to give the impression that a neurotic life is necessary for the investigator, but sometimes it helps.[3] Nor can we agree that the introverted personality is always interested in theory and the extravert in empirical research.

There is a curious but generalized attitude among investigators that seems like a continuation of the child's first attempts at mastery of the material world by practice in play. They playfully, with great pleasure, repeat actions many times until they can automatically perform them adequately. Scientists converse with each other by telling what they are "playing with now" or what is fun in their research. This also represents an outward minimization of the seriousness of their responsibilities for work and costs. But they are serious and sensitive to their sources of support, gaining relief by pretended unconcern.

In later life, during the formative years of professional education, the presence and influence of models of teachers who are engaged in research becomes tremendously important. They are significant at least for the beginning of an investigative career. It is from these models that the future researcher needs praise, encouragement and narcissistic gratification for his first efforts, no matter how futile they seem. Later rewards of increased prestige confirm the validity of his chosen efforts. If early sampling of research tasks gives rise to acceptable publication, the young investigator becomes "addicted" to more such success.

Yet during the course of his research he needs great patience and the ability to delay gratification because modern sophisticated clinical research requires huge amounts of time. Only few periods of serious researches are not monotonous because they require repetitive observations and experiments. It is during this period between closure of the research design and the final unanalyzed results that serendipity becomes important; that is, watching for the unexpected or unplanned that may be more important than the originally stated goals.

Benedek[4] states that scientific production reflects the personality of the scientist who creates something out of nothing (negentrophy). His own free associations plus a reflection of his own experiences gives him a glow of discovery, which must then be objectified by empirical studies. Such a capacity is a potential for creativity freed from preconcious processes that hold him within the confines of existing concepts.

A recent GAP report[5] contrasts the differential features of therapist and investigator. The former makes use of conventional wisdom, offers specific ameliorative action and thinks implicitly, vaguely and flexibly. The investigator, on the other hand, challenges conventional wisdom, understands general propositions and thinks in terms of explicit models linked to observable data.

Offer, Freedman[6] write:

> The investigator's professional qualifications, the auspices under which research is conducted, the subject studied, and the audience to whom the research is communicated are all factors in the general identification of researchers in psychiatry. Further, the choice of methodology affects the investigator's acceptability as a psychiatric researcher and determines his status within the various subgroupings of the psychiatric

community. Indeed there now tends to be a careeristic view of the researcher that requires that he engage in skilled systematic inquiry, distinguishing him sharply from the gentleman scholar model, the clinician who is inquisitive and enjoys sharing his thoughts and perceptions.

The GAP report #65[7] indicates that there is an urgent need to shift the attitude of psychiatrists to a more scientific orientation. This should begin with early research experiences in medical school, research orientation, training and supervision in residency training programs and, for those most interested, in postresidency research career grants.

Nordbeck and Maini[8] believe that only personal and anecdotal material is available to determine the relation of the researcher to research. Problem identification and problem solving vary with the individual's potential creative ability, his personality, childhood experiences, earlier research experiences and depressive moments. Changes in the direction of research depend on openness to discussion and criticism, sudden new ideas and concentration or diffusion of time. The personality of the investigator involves his degree of self-confidence, frustration and stress tolerance, depressive tendencies and degree of emotional involvement in his work. He requires the ability to change or restructure his methods and goals, endure failure and success and emerge from periods of low activity or pauses in his work.

Shakow[9] states that the need for research in the behavioral sciences is continuous and unremitting. There is a primary search for new knowledge and a need to evaluate so-called existing knowledge. Whether the investigator subscribes to the medical model of psychiatry or to the socioeducational model, he needs to cooperate with other disciplines rather than engage in useless quarrels.

The investigator needs energy, perseverance and sound work habits to unleash his cognitive potential for creative products. Although there is a need for more fulltime investigators, occasional participation and supportive technical services are also necessary. Investigators require training and experience in real life problems and real clinical situations. They need to learn how to observe and report, how to avoid bias or countertransference and possess empathy for the disturbed human being. With all the necessary education, there is a need for the researcher to maintain his own individuality because a wide range of personalities will contribute to modifications of existing models.

Kubie[10] denotes the qualities necessary for a scientific career:

> Scientific investigation proceeds by a series of steps, but not in a fixed or rigid sequence. Each step casts the scientist in a different role which makes different demands on him. In one he must be an observer, who attempts to see clearly, and not through eyes which are colored by his own biases. In another he constructs theoretical hypotheses concerning the interactions among the items he observes. In still a third, he makes experiments in which he takes some fragment of what he has observed in nature and reproduces simultaneous variables. Thereupon he must observe this creature of his own making with an objectivity which approximates the objectivity with which he made his original observations. He must record these observations without bias, make fresh theoretical hypotheses concerning them, and retest them by fresh experiments. This new set of experiments again becomes the facsimile of a fragment of nature to be observed, theorized about and subjected to a new order of tests. Thereupon he must once again become an observer, once again climbing out of his own skin, divesting himself of his pride of authorship, looking upon his

mental progeny as though they were somebody else's
children to be observed and tested dispassionately.

In sum, we cannot predict who will become an investigator in psychiatry; a subject of inquiry that badly needs evaluation and more valid knowledge. Nor can we designate
who has the creative potential. But our task is to encourage
the potential researcher through early educational systems,
by creating appropriate models and by furnishing an environment conducive for the young psychiatrist to devote his
energies, full- or part-time, to furthering knowledge in the
field. Whether the results are good, bad or only imitative,
a certain percentage of such people will produce substance
of value.[11]

Yet Maimonides[12] warned:

> If anybody tells you in order to support his opinion (or
> theory) that he is in possession of proofs and evidence
> and that he saw things with his own eyes, you have to
> doubt him, even if he is an authority, accepted by great
> men, even if he is himself honest and virtuous. Inquire
> well into what he wants to prove to you. Do not allow
> your senses to be confused by his research and innova-
> tion. Think well, search, examine and try to under-
> stand the ways of nature which he claims to know. I
> advise you to examine critically the opinion of even
> such an authority and prominent sage as Galen.

The outlook however is not good. A recent survey of the
National Institute for Mental Health's attempts to produce
researchers in psychiatry tells a dismal story.[13] After many
years of financial support to develop career investigators,
it is estimated that only about 250 psychiatrists are now
engaged in serious research. Facilities in which to work,
models to imitate and tools to use seem to be insufficient.
It seems that training programs for any subspecialty (child,

family, group *and* research) require the selection of students whose life style has already fit them for their career choices. An investigator can be developed only if he is already prepared, which clearly indicates that developing future personnel for psychiatric research is a problem of selection.

REFERENCES

1. Roe, A. *The making of a scientist.* New York: Dodd Mead, 1953.
2. Bowlby, J. Attachment and loss. Vol. II. *Separation, anxiety and anger.* New York: Basic Books, 1970.
3. Kubie, L. S. *Neurotic distortion of the creative process.* Lawrence, Kan.: University of Kansas Press, 1958.
4. Benedek, T. *Psychoanalytic investigations: selected papers.* New York: Quandrangle New York Times Books, 1973.
5. Group for the Advancement of Psychiatry. Report #73: *Psychotherapy and the dual research tradition.* (Vol. II), 1969.
6. Offer, D., & Freedman, D. X. (Eds.) *Modern psychiatry and clinical research.* New York: Basic Books, 1972.
7. Group for the Advancement of Psychiatry. Report #65: *The recruitment and training of the research psychiatrist,* **543,** 1967.
8. Nordbeck, B., & Maini, S. M. Psychology of the researcher and research. *Psychological research bulletin of Lund University,* (Sweden) 1970, **10, 11.**
9. Shakow, D. The education of the mental health researcher. *Arch. Gen. Psychiatry,* 1972, **27,** 15–25.
10. Kubie, L. S. Research in psychiatry. Problems in training experience and strategy. In H. W. Brosin (Ed.), *Lectures on experimental psychiatry.* Pittsburgh: University of Pittsburgh Press, 1959.
11. Kaplan, A. *The conduct of inquiry.* San Francisco: Chandler, 1964.
12. Maimonides 1135–1204. Cited in S. J. Zakon, *Medica Judaica,* 1971, **1,** 16–21.
13. Boothe, B. E., Rosenfeld, A. H., & Walker, E. R.: *Toward a science of psychiatry: impact of the research development of the national institute of mental health.* Monterey, Calif.: Wadsworth Publishing Co., 1974.

V

The Object of Inquiry in Psychiatry

It has often been repeated that one has to ask the right questions in order to reach reliable and valid answers. It seems strange in this modern world that we still argue over the fundamental question: what is psychiatry? Since World War II, psychiatry has become one of the five major fields of study in medical schools and in the large teaching hospitals. Even before World War II—in fact for about the last 100 years—psychiatry has been defined as the medical specialty concerned with the medical practice or applied science of diagnosing, treating and preventing mental diseases or disorders of the mind.[1]

It seems more appropriate today to consider Masserman's[2] broader pluralistic definition: "Psychiatry can be broadly defined as a *science* which deals with the determining factors of human behavior, its variations and vicissitudes, the methods of its analysis, and the means that may be employed to align behavior with optimal personal and social goals." The differences between these two definitions indicate that profound changes have taken place over the last decades. We shall consider psychiatry as a science in this chapter, and forgo further and perhaps finer defini-

69

tions of the term until after we have considered in a later chapter, health and normality.

We are thus confronted with the question, What kind of a science is psychiatry? It is not like the "hard" sciences of physics and mathematics, but changes with the Zeitgeist, or ways of viewing the world, since it is a study of interbehaviors,[3] individuals, societies and cultures. As a science, psychiatry cannot fall back on philosophy or the supernatural but requires rigorous testing and investigations.[4]

Both lay people and professional psychiatrists continue to view psychiatry in its limited role as a therapeutic branch of medicine—an applied science. In so doing, psychiatry is considered to be a conglomerate of various therapeutic techniques. As a matter of fact, no hard facts have been derived from the few investigations and follow-up studies of various methods of treatment. The many kinds of individual, family, group and community therapies of ancient and current times give no indication of specific therapy for special circumstances. Logic would dictate that the therapies all involve a nonspecific goal for helping people in trouble, an empathy for their misery and a respect for their humanity.

How then do we view our present society's system of psychotherapeutic activities? In terms of the available evidence relating to social system input (especially patient demography and client institutions), it begins to appear that the major de facto function of our therapeutic activity system is *as a kind of higher education in the development of interpersonal skills and emotional capacities.* It parallels the function of collegiate education, in which occupational skills and instrumental capacities are developed to the high level required by our socioeconomic system. Those who have higher education in the latter sphere frequently also find a need for it in the former. Personal distress is still a critical factor in determining a person's becoming a patient in psychotherapy, but it is distress (or aberrant reactions to stress) occasioned by experienced frustration or failure in social-emotional functioning, rather than distress occasioned by (somatic) illness. Psychotherapeutic "education" is tutorial in form, and often requires remedial work to correct dysfunctional interpersonal and emotional patterns learned in the course of family and peer group socialization, but it characteristically includes more advanced work as well such as intimacy, spontaneity, self-disclosure, etc.[5]

Strupp[6] emphasizes in general the fact that the patient develops trust in the therapist's authority and control. The several successful techniques indicate the absence of a specific scientific model. The core of psychiatry is often held to consist of the ability to communicate about the here and now with one other person in a dyadic system. We have learned through experiences ballooned by enthusiasms and crushed by disappointments that psychiatry is much more. We believe it far clearer to use the term "transactions;" that is, an umbrella term under which the setting and purpose, the overt and covert language, the reverberating and spiraling processes and the techniques of altering the system of communications are defined.[7] These processes are demonstrated in the transactions between patients and therapists in various settings.

We now know that we should approach living human beings as if they exist in a total field of multiple transactions. Thereby we avoid the dichotomies of nature *vs.* nurture, organic *vs.* functional, lower *vs.* higher or reduction *vs.* extension. Furthermore, we can then deal operationally with multivariable problems from a stance that really takes into account the multicausality of both healthy and disordered function. This is transactionalism in a total field whose constituents range from physicochemical to symbolic foci. Opponents of this broad concept are exclusively specialized therapists who contend that such an approach dilutes or weakens dynamic psychotherapy.

These dynamic approaches within a dyad have frequently resulted in a depreciation of the basic psychiatric scientific techniques through which much progress was made in the nineteenth century. These are the methods of careful unbiased and controlled observations and accurate descriptions of behavior-over-time, including verbalizations, but not limited to them. Observation of behavior rather than inferences about feelings is the keystone of psychiatric research. Actually, behavior represents functions allocated to an hypothetical ego which filters perceptions on the one hand and actions on the other, which expresses reportable motivations, affects, defenses and compromises, which employs symptoms and sublimations and demonstrates integrative capacities and disintegrative trends. About any of these there need be few primary inferences or interpretations. As observational material they can be coded, rated, replicated and tracked through time. These basic living data can *then* be interpreted according to their validation or disproof of any hypothesis. In addition, information gained from "depth" interviews may account for deviances and interindividual variability, but the behaviors of the participant-observer and of the subject whose "internal behaviors" are being observed, as in psychoanalytic sessions, require adequate systems of recording of data and their subsequent analysis. The acquisition and validity-testing of behavioral data are the core operations of psychiatry as a science.

Feigl[8] states that scientists seek descriptions, explanation and predictions which are as adequate and accurate as possible. "Instead of presenting a finished account of the world, the genuine scientist keeps his unifying hypotheses open to revision and is always ready to modify or abandon them if evidence should render them doubtful." Feigl's basic assumption is that empirical science is an unending quest for knowledge and that its claims to truth are never absolute, but are always held open to correction, verification or disproof; and, therefore, scientific truths differ only in degree from knowledge accumulated throughout the ages by sound common sense. The quest for scientific truth is, however, a unique process in that it is regulated by certain standards or criteria which are best formulated as ideals to be approximated, rather than as goals ever fully attained. According to Feigl, it is a sign of maturity to be able to live with an unfinished world view.

Kaplan[9] states that the behavioral sciences (excluding psychiatry) are overloaded by theories and their proliferation. A good theory is one worth being acted on in contexts of inquiry or of other action. Theory is true if it fits the facts, if predictions made on the basis of theory are in fact fulfilled, but not if the facts are wholly constituted by the theory they are adduced to support and if they lack an operational core. The value of a theory is not only in the answers it gives, but in new questions it raises.

Since early antiquity, mental diseases have been classified from various frames of reference which Menninger[10] has laboriously collected. It is not our purpose to review these many systems included in the Science of Systematics since the time of Aristotle. Currently there exists a useless controversy regarding diagnoses, despite the Dewey and Bentley[11] axiom: "Naming is knowing." Modern classifications began in the 18th and 19th centuries, culminating in Kraepelin's classification system based on outcome and specifying cause, course and end result. During the century, this system has been modified, though only slightly, to correspond with a more sophisticated outlook; although even now, nineteenth-century single-causes and linear phenomena have not perished. Obviously we cannot write a textbook on the various accepted names of syndromes. Schools, geographical areas, countries, etc. have different names and definitions. Our purpose is to state quite simply that diagnosis is the primary question with which psychiatric research must deal.

During most of the first half of the twentieth century, research in psychiatry was unsystematic and unorganized, as is characteristic of a young science. Astute clinical psychiatrists made observations on disturbances that seemed new and different from those they had known heretofore, and they published these observations in current periodicals. Few advances were made and little new knowledge was acquired by this method.

After World War II, when funds were available in 1946 from the National Institute of Mental Health, even good applications submitted to the Research Study Group were rejected because qualified personnel were not available. Only after training grants for psychiatric residents became effective—grants that were distributed to medical schools and other training centers throughout the country—did some graduates became interested in research on psychiatric problems. But these were all too few. Despite our warnings of the pitfalls of a full-time practice career, many graduates devoted their whole professional lives either to private practice or, at the most, to part-time positions in institutional treatment clinics.

Often these practitioners became bored with their monotonous work and in middle life approached us with a desire to "Do some research." What did they want to do? The usual answer was that they did not know and expected to be assigned to a project or to latch onto an existing program. With little preparation, low motivation, and no concept of the scientific method despite their extensive clinical experiences, their requests had to be denied. Or the best of these bored psychiatrists started a borrowed project which they never completed.

There are three standard questions that must be asked by any of the disciplines in the life sciences, including the science of psychiatry. These are: what, how and why? The abstractions, among others, pertain to the object of inquiry in our field. The "what" refers specifically to definition of nosological entities in our currently confused system of classification.[12] The "how" focuses on the multiple causes and the interrelations between them that are specific to each clinical syndrome. The "why" questions the adaptive or maladaptive values or effects of each type of disturbance.

Despite many therapists, especially psychotherapists and psychoanalysts, who state that they are only interested in their individual patients and do not care about diagnosis, psychiatry could never be a science without a system of diagnostic classification. Within the classes of psychoses, neuroses and personality disorders are many subdivisions characterized by similarities and differences from other subdivisions. Such systems of naming are the basis of the medical model of psychiatry that began with Hippocrates followed by gradual evolution and clarification by philosophers and psychologists.

Kraepelin first combined various dementias into Dementia Praecox, now known as Schizophrenia, and then in 1899 developed a comprehensive diagnostic system. This persisted over many decades and naming became a primary objective of "State Hospital" psychiatrists. Although the American system of classification has been altered every 10 years and it now follows the International Classification, it is beset with many errors of the past continuously carried over to the present. Definitions are so vague that psychiatric diagnoses vary from school to school, from area to area and country to country. Furthermore, our system of classification has not accounted for the changing characteristics of the neuroses and psychoses.[13] The deficiencies of the system have hindered progress and needs to be overhauled in order to answer the question "what." But to state that diagnoses are irrevelant and should be abolished because mental disturbances are problems in living, only alleviated by changing our society, is a regressive rather than a progressive move and is not even a valid psychosocial model.

One GAP Report[14] makes the following statement:

> The research psychiatrist is expected to make a special contribution to behavioral science because of a unique perspective from clinical training and experience. As a physician he assumes medical responsibility in research involving human subjects. Medical training emphasizes the application of the basic biological sciences to clinical problems. From clinical study and practice, the psychiatrist has gained first-hand knowledge of mental disorders, from minor maladjustments to severe psychoses. He examines a clinical situation in its full complexity, with awareness of significant factors in the patient's biological functioning, personal development, family relationships, and cultural setting. Psychiatrists are needed both to design research on the problems of clinical psychiatry and to bring to behavioral research the issues and techniques of psychiatry.

Millon and Diesenhaus[15] state that a given individual's interest in psychiatric research may be attributed to several factors. The psychiatrist may be curious about a particular issue or be doubtful and skeptical about a certain assumption. He may choose to investigate a particular subject because current popularity makes it expedient or practical. Hypotheses are chosen from previous empirical findings bolstered by specified assumptions and oriented toward one of the biophysical, intrapsychic, phenomenological or sociocultural levels or, at best, some form of bridging among these levels.[16]

The focus of research in psychiatry, then, is whatever society and culture determine to be disturbed or deviant behavior and/or a class, subgroup or individual person who feels badly even though his behavior does not directly reveal his state of mind. Thus research focuses on cognition, affects, perceptions and behaviors. The term behavior is a generalization including not only gross total or global and verbal behaviors, but also physiological and biochemical actions.[3]

The investigator may focus on the unfolding maturational processes, the development dependent on life experiences or so-called stresses, on early or later somatic accidents (diseases or trauma), on family characteristics or on rapidly changing social and cultural conditions. Research is necessary in the area of conflicts, defenses and coping devices and interpersonal transactions dependent on capacities to assume appropriate roles.

If the potential investigator has acquired sufficient clinical experience he will have plenty of opportunity to doubt, to be skeptical and to be curious. Some of the hitches in our field may stimulate the most creative individuals to develop new paradigms.[17] In addition one focus may lead the investigator into other disciplines; for which he can obtain the help he needs by establishing a multidisciplinary group. For example, clinical studies on types of depression lead to family studies, genetics and biochemistry. All of these disciplines become necessary elements in ferreting out the answer to the "what" question and leading to some information about "how."

The investigator should know that research may be divided in general by focus or method. Ideographic research applies to observations on individual cases; a research system that has become increasingly unproductive. Nomothetic research searches for general laws of thinking, feeling and behaviors. Likewise, deductive research depends on theory and general assumptions applied to specific cases, while inductive research begins with empirical data from which general principles concerning classes of the above are derived.

In all these researches, mathematical or statistical applications may be essential but not to the exclusion of other forms of study. For example, counting "stress situations" prior to and leading up to physical or mental illness in an effort thereby to predict the time of onset, severity and duration of illness is only one part of a total system. Research also requires including studies of personality types and the quality and meaning of those situations which provoke "stress responses"—including the stress response of successful coping.

Anyone entering into the research field has many options from which to choose the object of his inquiry. He may do empirical or analytic "sorting," which is badly needed given our present state in which diseases, disturbances or syndromes are poorly defined. He may study processes of integration or regulation and systematize relationships. Whatever his choice, he is required to define his goals, for these are the bases of levels of operation and methods of procedure.

He may wish to accumulate knowledge through empirical methods of observation or experimentation about a particular entity—the so-called "target" or "mission" research that is now favored by granting agents. But whatever his objective, he must recognize that he has built-in biases that are characteristic of his own lifestyle and system of values.

To avoid hit or miss, trivial or repetitive research, an investigator should make a literature search. This may help him choose clinically significant problems and avoid the "me too" results. Any new information regarding classification of aberrant behavior cannot be confused with causes that answer the question "how." Nor should he too quickly jump to what Herrick calls "respectable teleology," the "why" question; that is, the adaptive functions of the disturbance.

Finally, research begins with assumptions or models used as test hypotheses but necessarily based on prior knowledge and experience in the field. Then observations are made on the basis of active choice, but which have some relationship to the goal of the research. Even with the greatest of care, observations are never complete nor free from distortions.

REFERENCES

1. Grinker, R. R., Sr. Identity or regression in American psychoanalysis. *Arch. Gen. Psych,* 1965, **12,** 113–125.
2. Masserman, J. H. *Principles of dynamic psychiatry.* (2nd. ed.) New York: W. B. Saunders, 1961.
3. Kantor, J. R. *Scientific evolution of psychology.* Granville, Ohio: Principia Press, 1963.
4. Langer, S. *Philosophy in a new key.* Cambridge, Mass.: Harvard University Press, 1942.
5. Howard, K. I., & Orlinsky, D. E. Psychotherapeutic process. *Annual Review of Psychology,* 1972, **23,** 615–668.
6. Strupp, H. H. Specific *vs* nonspecific factors in psychotherapy and the problem of control. *Arch. Gen. Psych,* 1970, **23,** 393–401.
7. Grinker, R. R., Sr., MacGregor, H., Selan, K., Klein, A., & Kohrman, J. *Psychiatric social work: a transactional case-book.* New York: Basic Books, 1961.
8. Feigl, H. & Brodbeck, M. (Eds.) *Readings in philosophy of science.* New York: Appleton-Century-Crofts, 1953.
9. Kaplan, A. *The Conduct of inquiry.* San Francisco: Chandler, 1964.
10. Menninger, K. *The vital balance.* New York: Viking, 1963.
11. Dewey, J. & Bentley, A. F. *Knowing and the known.* Boston: Beacon Press, 1949.
12. Hoch, P. H. *Differential diagnosis in clinical psychiatry.* New York: Science House, 1972.
13. Schimel, J. L., Salzman, L., Chodoff, P. L., Grinker, R. R., Sr., & Will, O. Changing styles in psychiatric syndromes: a symposium. *Amer. J. Psychiatry,* 1973, **130,** 147–155.
14. Group for the Advancement of Psychiatry. Report #65: *The recruitment and training of the research psychiatrist,* **543,** 1967.

15. Millon, T, & Diesenhaus, H. I. *Research methods in psychopathology.* New York: John Wiley, 1972.
16. Offer, D., Freedman, D. X. & Offer, J. L. (Eds.) *Modern psychiatry and clinical research.* New York: Basic Books, 1972.
17. Kuhn, T. S. *Structure of scientific revolutions.* Chicago: University of Chicago Press, 1962.

VI

Research Designing

Psychiatry, or psychopathology, is no longer considered a field exclusively concerned with medicine or psychology; it is now recognized to include four areas of data: biophysical, intrapsychic, phenomenological and behavioral—each representing a different perspective and using different methods.[1] Hopefully, some day these areas may be integrated. At present, methods—as, for example, exploration, description and confirmation—are aims in themselves that have distinguishing characteristics.[2]

To begin with, in order to develop hypotheses, we need a system of classification of psychiatric entities; entities which have by no means been sharply defined. This requirement demands systematic empirical observations based on specific protocols designed for the problem to be solved. Yet, even theoretical speculations, so long as they are used explicitly to build models, may lead to good empirical research if sharp operational definitions are then developed. Finally, hypothetical constructs and the use of unknown but intervening variables may be temporarily employed. Thus various types of research may result in so-called hard *or* speculative results.

There are other ways to delineate psychiatric research than in terms of the traditional categories of inductive or deductive; these include ideographic (individual) and nomothetic (study of classes) studies. We may use naturalistic *or* experimental research, each with its own design, technique and kinds of results. Transactional research presupposes that all behaviors change in time, and refers to what changes occur and, perhaps, how they occur. There are, however, limits to experimentation with humans, so that the naturalistic method in a free field furnishes the maximum freedom for either cross-sectional short-term or longitudinal, long-term research. These two methods have different degrees of flexibility or tightness of closure.[3]

We are interested in developing a general theory that applies to both health and illness. Such a theory would have particular reference to ontological or developmental processes as applied to health, and to etiology as applied to disease. A systematic way of relating the medical sciences to the life cycle of health and disease could also appropriately contribute to a logical organization of medical education.

It is quite apparent that, when we consider the growth and development of the human organism, we can observe an increasing individuality. It might be summarized by stating that developed man, despite his stages or levels of order, represents processes of irreducible logical complexities. This means that education about man, as contrasted with the lower animals, must be modified to include the complexities that accentuate individuality.[4]

Genetics or constitution, heredity, etc. are the givens with which an organism is born, yet—and this is the basic assumption of the ethologists—the genetic background cannot manifest itself except through transactions with environmental releasing mechanisms. Furthermore, genetic processes are not only apparent to some degree at birth, but influence the *entire* process of development, including the character and timing of aging and death. Thus the genetic framework maintains its influence during all of life.

On the other hand, environments consisting of social and cultural processes are also limiting factors. Environmental factors are presumed to be relatively constant, if one considers the social and cultural "surround" within a civilization as a *general* process, not including the specific ethnic and social groups which we will discuss later. However, the environment as an "invariant" is slowly changing through social and cultural evolution, and rapidly changing through revolutionary upheaval. Thus, the student revolution in the colleges and the civil rights revolution have been effective in changing the entire socio-cultural environment of our nation.

We *begin* with the relatively undifferentiated infant who is born with a particular genetic background and into a particular society and culture. As a relatively undifferentiated organism, its genetic potentialities are only partially revealed by morphological states. Genetic variations such as potentialities or drive strengths can only be surmised by the degree of activity and the complexity of the random motor movements of the infant. Many secretory and endocrine differences of genetic origin are only manifested when the organism is challenged in life.

The *second* stage is one of considerable differentiation in which the organism has now incorporated within its psychosomatic systems memory traces derived from its experiences in a particular environment. Thus, the mother/child relations, the father/child relations, the child/child relations, the child/school, the child/church—all these relationships, plus experiences in the family as a unit, and in many other groups, serve to differentiate the organism. The internalized experiences which become the subsystems may not at this stage all be fully developed, but they eventually contribute to the degree of homeostatic effectiveness within the organism. Thus, if a mother/child relationship is defective, child/peer relationship may compensate for that later.

Differentiation in this stage is based upon cognitive, emotional and physical learning. These learning systems may consist of reinforcement of conditioned reflexes, of mechanisms that release innate properties, of imitation and, by incorporating memory images of both psychic and somatic experiences, of so-called identifications.

The *third* phase is the life style of the individual as expressed in adolescence. It includes his somatic behavior, his personality and his coping devices which are specific for him and remain relatively constant. It is sometimes said that new defensive devices can sometimes only be learned by the developed "self system" later in life. As a matter of fact, it seems improbable that by stages two or three there can be much reversibility or change in the phenotypes.

The *fourth* stage is more appropriate to young adult life, and is characterized by varying degrees of health and varying degrees of proneness to disintegration or disease. The proneness or susceptibility requires suitable environmental agencies to result in an overt state of sickness. Health, however, may persist in a relative sense until the next phase.

The *fifth* phase consists of the stages of aging, with the disease or illness that is characteristic of the processes of wearing down. Disease really means dis-ease or uncomfortableness, an expression of the effect a particular environmental influence has on the organism developed to this stage of life, influenced as it has been by its past experiences and its genetic background. In chronic illness, the disease-state manifests itself without much shift. The acute phase may be transient and reversible to the premorbid condition, but lesser degrees of reversibility are possible in the process of aging.

In a *later* phase the person who has assumed a career as a patient has only a future in dying and death.

One can diagram this series of events in the form of a semicircle in relation to gravity. Thus, the infant struggles against gravity and gradually moves upright into the erect posture of the adult. Slowly as he gets older he moves down again and finally gravity wins out and he is leveled to the ground. Of course, there are short-cuts to this phase of dying and death, which can occur in any phase of development. The schizophrenic might say that the lifecycle is a painful journey from the womb to the tomb, so he chooses not to go through the vicissitudes of life and makes a direct journey by suicide.

The characteristics of this system of analysis indicate that in growth and development, the trend is upward from relative undifferentiation to differentiation. There are also processes which force the organism back to a more undifferentiated state. This is perhaps more easily understandable when we speak of psychological regression, but it does occur as well in physical regression.

If we view this method of analysis of the human system, it is apparent that each individual system—that is, each human being—is itself composed of subsystems of variables. Each system is a combination of genetic and environmental factors, the latter contributing to experience, learning and coping. Each system is related to the other stages of the life cycle. When we realize that there are no sharp dichotomies between genetics and environment and no absolute differentiation between levels of development and that no phase of the lifecycle is independent, I think that we will have accomplished what might be called the philosophy of ontology in relation to scientific disciplines and to the therapeutic aspects of medicine.

There are many scientific disciplines contributing to our knowledge of mental health and illness, including psychopharmacology, psychoanalysis and dynamic models, existential concepts, epidemiology, biometrics and probably more.[5] Since each has a voluminous literature of books and periodicals, even abstracting them would require several encyclopedias. We shall, therefore, in the chapters that follow, delineate some significant research questions and some methods in capsule form. In the meantime, we ought not to forget some of the practical difficulties involved in research:

Sophistication in clinical psychiatric investigations demands incredible amounts of time, energy and money, so attention must be given, before the project or program is begun, to the various steps or parts of these procedures and to their overall organization.

Research is not conducted in a vacuum. Except for the old-fashioned introspective technique utilized in the past by some schools of psychology and psychiatry, clinical research requires a physical setting conducive to interviews, observations, tests and questionnaires. This includes a private room for interviewing and one-way screens for observations of behavior of individuals, groups and families. Also, observations of subject-behavior in the free-field of a nursing unit exposes social interactions.

The human environment, or what we may term the atmosphere in which the research is to be conducted, depends largely on the character and interests of the chairman of the department. He can hinder or facilitate the work of an investigator and even serve as a model for him. So, for example, he may make time available for the clinician's research activities, liberate him from administrative tasks and free him from obstructing administrative controls. There should be an autonomy of inquiry.

The investigator, with the help of the chairman, usually has to interest and inspire cooperating and participating personnel. The paid assistants and technicians usually present no problem, but the noninvolved clinicians may obstruct or sabotage the utilization of their patients, private or service, for whom they are the physicians-of-record. The problem is one of education. As Offer and Freedman[5] state:

> It is precisely the advancement of this pattern of practice, reflection, investigation, and communication in

psychiatry that is really meant when we focus on the practical issues of advancing research in departments of psychiatry. Though the literature reviewed might well be applicable to the behavioral sciences generally, and though we are vitally interested in the relevance of related biobehavioral sciences, our explicit emphasis here is on psychiatrists themselves working in research and the importance of this for sound growth of the discipline. The fact is that it is the scholarly or research-minded psychiatrist who must introduce his clinical colleagues to developments occuring outside the confines of the discipline. We need psychiatrists who acquire the special competencies necessary for rendering such translations less corrupted and banal than they often have been. This bridging work should also make findings from other areas more readily and soundly applicable to the core interests of psychiatry.

Many clinicians are strictly therapeutic specialists within a department of psychiatry. They refuse to cooperate, and especially they refuse to lend their patients for harmless procedures about which they are fully informed. As Anthony[6] states, child psychiatrists seem even more obstructive than most:

> There are many clinicians whose experience of the NIMH granting propensities have been such that they are ready to condemn all contemporary research in the field of psychiatry (especially that done by non-psychiatrists) as trivial and given to methodology. They will warn residents against premature engagement in research before they have acquired adequate clinical background and experience. They will sneer at findings that are no more than elephantine gleams into the obvious. . . . It is also well for the researcher to remember (and, in fact, fatal for him to forget) that for many of them, there is something vaguely threatening about research. They may see it as intrusive,

intimidating, dehumanizing and fixated on numbers. Perhaps, its greatest crime in their eyes lies in approaching children in a non-therapeutic way and perceiving them in terms of means and not ends. This would imply an absence of alliances, of working through and of respect for defenses. The patient loses his identity and becomes a figure among other figures and, following the statistical analysis, he is no longer considered to exist. There is no responsibility for him and no concern about his future except in follow-up studies.

The questions for investigations cover a wide area since so much is unknown and needs researching. An incomplete list of these questions will be suggested later. It is more important at this point to propose some generalizations, the first of which concerns the interest, commitment and real involvement of the investigator. The absence of real motivation or pressure to do a particular task or to join a particular program or project, rarely results in completion of the work or a satisfactory outcome. The question for research must arise from the researcher himself. Empirical research is lengthy and hard work.

Many investigators choose problems that are currently fashionable and hop on the most available bandwagon, or use readily available methods (Kaplan's[7] law of the instrument), thereby producing only repetitive or imitative "me too" conclusions; or he may latch onto existing programs because they are already organized and defined.

A mundane and somewhat corrupt practice develops when the investigator decides to work on problems that may not interest him greatly, but for which supporting money is available; it is like the bank robber who, when asked why he robs banks, answered, "because that's where the money is." Increasingly, the governmental funding agents are interested in supporting research that is directly relevant to human problems—the so-called "mission oriented" research. The fallacy of avoiding basic research has been discussed many times, and examples are often given of how seemingly unrelated laboratory research may become practical and pertinent to human disease. This holds true whether the research is problem- or method-oriented, exploratory or focused on a specific life-destroying disease.

One of the most serious problems in clinical research in psychiatry, where so many variables exist and seem to cry out for consideration, is the tendency initially to include too much data, without focusing on the material meaningful to the particular problem. One cannot study everything at one time. It is necessary to be content with small parts of the total system, well-described subsystems, or pay the price of becoming inundated with indigestible numbers. The analogy is pertinent because tyros come to the research table wanting to take in too much. "Their eyes are bigger than their stomachs." Yet it does take courage to face research seminars and professional meetings and hear so many questions beginning with: "Why didn't you_____?"

Before proceeding in the orderly development of investigations, the researcher should recognize the theory, based on clear assumptions, under which he will operate. He then may extract his hypothesis and clearly define his dependent and independent variables, for which he needs information and experience. Without these his questions will flounder in a sea of uncertainty and he will founder on the rocks of trivia.

Using psychotherapy as an example, Sargent[8] generalized about the relation between the theories leading to research questions and the kinds of data which should be sought:

> If, within the behavioral context, psychotherapy is regarded as a matter of learning and conditioning, out-

come will be measured in terms of learned adaptations. If it is conceived of as a special case of social interaction, or of communication, change in interpersonal variables will be sought. If increased conscious comfort and self-acceptance are seen as the primary therapeutic goals, self-descriptions of feelings states will be prominent in the data. If theory recognizes such constructs as the ego, in which reorganization may come about with or without direct or immediate reflection in verbal report or behavior, dynamic balances and ego functions become the variables of interest, and methods suited to their study are needed.

She agrees with the model "behavior-observation-inference," and that good theory implies methods for confirmation, as good methods are sired by theory. Then, when the investigator knows what he wants to do, he should know what has already been done.[9] Even though he may be a mature clinician, well-trained and knowledgeable, he should not fail to consult primary sources—taking nothing for granted—and he should check everything, including bibliographies in other fields. Nevertheless, he needs to avoid being inundated with pottering material or overwhelmed by minutiae.

Then it is necessary to place his acquired informations in proper context in relation to his problem, and to utilize them in his discriminating judgment. He can then more clearly specify the phenomena to be studied. Knowing what has been done he may avoid simple repetition, and his critique of prior research can help him avoid the pitfalls of his own. A good example is the huge number of papers and books published on schizophrenia, which use every conceivable technique but never come to grips with what that entity is that we call schizophrenia. Messy psychiatric nosology and classification have ruined many investigators.

The next step is to plan a design involving methods and techniques pertinent to the problem. These must fit the specified questions. Planning may involve the single investigator through his own cognitive processes, or it may involve thorough discussions with research groups. If the research group is multidisciplinary, common, easily understood, agreed-on definitions must be developed from the different jargons.

Each member of the group should have his responsibilities allocated and the activities of each person or discipline should be carefully scheduled. A whole set of investigators cannot attack the research subject at the same time. Simultaneity of measurements, although desirable, is only approximate. Also, if correlations are to be made using different approaches, contaminations must be avoided to prevent investigators influencing each other by prior knowledge of the other's results.

Finally, in the planning stage, discussions tend to be repetitive and interminable. There often seems to be reluctance to start the work, which everyone knows will be arduous, and discussions, while not as productive, may be more exciting and educational. The principal investigator finally has to state: "Now we start." It may be premature, but that is a calculated risk.

In this world of ethical confusion and dubiety, because some investigators have violated basic ethical considerations in working with human subjects, each research center now by law has to set up a review committee to review its research projects. The federal law makes the following specifications:

Advisory committees are required in their consideration of proposals to determine whether the rights and welfare of human subjects will be adequately protected. Therefore, if the protocol involves human subjects as defined by policy, the principal investigator shall include under the heading human subjects at the end of the *Methods of Procedure* section of the application: (1) an assessment of any physical, psychological, sociological, or other risks or possible detrimental effects of the planned work, and an assessment of the benefits to be gained by the individual subject as well as benefits which will accrue to society in general as a result of the planned work; (2) an analysis of the "risk-benefit ratio" and (3) a description of the measures to be taken to protect the rights of subjects, including criteria for the selection of subjects and the planned procedures to obtain informed consent.*

When planning is at least tentatively completed, the next step is the pilot study. In this phase, the chosen design is pretested by engaging in one or more sets of observation and experimentation. It may be considered as a "dry run," leading in many cases to a modification of the design. Sometimes some observational or experimental techniques will have to be added, but most often some will be omitted as redundant, too ambitious or not relevant to the central problem. We tend to start out by including too many variables that we cannot control.

It is wise at this tentative stage to include the person who will be involved in statistical analysis of the data, if the goal involves quantities. He will advise how feasible an analysis of results will be and advise on numbers needed, methods of denotation and coding techniques for programming and computer analysis. It is better to do this earlier rather than later because many times, after great labor, the statistician cannot be of help. His disgust then expresses itself in the cliché, "Garbage in—garbage out."

Usually the pilot or pretest study in clinical psychiatry will reveal that old and current hospital records are not utilizable because they have been written at various times

*As cited in John Romano's essay: Reflections on Informed Consent. *Archives of General Psychiatry*, 1974, **30**, 129–135.

by many different residents and students. The contents of such records are uneven, omitting notations that are essential for the clinical research. For this reason it is advisable to begin with a clinical protocol specially devised and suitable for each project.

Another difficulty that becomes apparent in the pilot study is the vagueness and inaccuracy of retrospective data. The subject may not remember or may be reluctant to reveal his past. Likewise, the parents of subject children frequently indulge in retrospective falsification. These obstacles require interviews with a series of informants in order to develop a reasonably accurate consensus.

Data collection depends naturally on the research methods employed and should be guided by statistical advice. Even so, hitches are frequently encountered that require modification of the design for the full-scale research that follows the pilot study. This is why the design should not be locked prematurely and should not be too tightly organized at the cost of flexibility. A high percentage of research endeavors fail for this and similar reasons, when hitches cannot be overcome and data are irrelevant to the purpose of the research. These failures are rarely reported. When the experienced and often renowed investigator recounts how he proceeded from results to new hypotheses in an uninterrupted straight line, he is not being truthful, and he also discourages the young aspiring investigator who is made to feel inferior.

There are a number of words that indicate that an observer or experimenter, especially in the behavioral sciences, is not completely objective. As Kaplan states, he is never free of ideational elements.[7] We call him biased, emotionally committed to positive results, constricted by his own personality or suffering from countertransference intrusions. These phenomena come down to his faith in his goals or his humanitarian stance. Science has attempted to counteract these trends by tests of reliability. This simply means that other members of the team or outsiders not associated with the research independently judge the data, or that tests or observations are repeated. This requires that each such person speak and understand the same language and is in tune with the definitions of each item. Without such preparation, tests of reliability are a waste of time. For purposes of concise data collection and for reliability, it is necessary to employ scaling devices in well-conceived rating systems and codification.

If reliability of observation is important in psychiatric research, we must ask: what are the conditions under which independent agreement among judges is most likely to be achieved? (Hamburg *et al.*[10]). While this problem has had very little attention in the psychiatric literature, it has been taken more seriously in the related fields of psychology and sociology. Bruner and Tagiuri[11] have recently reviewed a large literature on the recognition of emotions and the judgment of personality characteristics. They have called attention to four major technical problems that affect the reliable observation of emotional and personality variables:

1. *The nature of the discrimination required in an emotion-judging task.* They point out that it is more difficult to distinguish one unpleasant emotional state from another unpleasant one than it is to distinguish love and disgust. In other words, the difficulty of the task is one important factor that determines the reliability of observation.

2. *The nature of the identifying labels the judges are asked to use.* Outside judges reach higher agreement in judging if they are not allowed to use their own terminology and categories. There is no reason to assume that different individuals are equally inclined to utilize the same categories for ordering emotional expression.

3. *Adequacy of information.* This seems to be a particularly important point. The accuracy of judgment appears to be directly related to the amount of informations given the observer. Each item of relevant information narrows the

range of likely alternatives. In general, then, "the more information about the situation in which an emotion is being expressed, the more accurate and reliable are judgments of the emotions."

4. *The problem of sampling emotional expressions.* There is a great variability in the ways used by different subjects to express the same emotion. Indeed, there is even some variability in the ways in which a given subject expresses a given emotion at different times. Therefore, it is important to have a rather wide sampling of expressions for each subject, and for the population of subjects from which a given subject is drawn. Both for crosscultural and intracultural reasons, it is quite unwise to assume a stereotyped set of behavior as the required expression for a given emotion. The observers must, if they are to make reliable estimates, know a good deal about each subject and about the type of subject he represents.

In a similar review, Heynes and Lippitt[12] come to three main conclusions about conditions which influence the reliability of observation in studies of human behavior:

1. *Degree of inference.* The less inference required of observers, the higher the degree of agreement. With category or rating systems which require a good deal of inference, it is clear that the most reliable are those in which the dimensions are clearly defined and the cues to be used by the observers are specified.

2. *Definition of the unit of observation.* The reliability of some systems is low because of unclear definition of the unit. Even when the units to be rated or classified may be fairly clearly stated, the observers may nevertheless disagree as to unit boundaries in actual observing situations. It is obvious that the degree of agreement as to coding can only be appropriately assessed when there is agreement first as to what is to be coded.

3. *Training of observers.* With category or rating systems which require some inference, the degree of reliability attained is very much a function of the amount of training which observers have had. The thoroughly trained observer has become maximally familiar with the definitions of the categories or dimensions. He has gotten practice in designating the unit of observation. He has gained skill in adopting the frame of reference which the system demands, and has practiced his art in the situation in which the behavior takes place. His own private definitions have been eliminated or have come to be shared using the system. In short, virtually all the sources of unreliability have been dealt with in the training.

We shall not discuss here the statistical methods of data analysis. These highly sophisticated processes require the services of specialized persons. The statistician will have been prepared to use appropriate methods for the kind of data acquired, although he has many possible maneuvers depending on the results. He expresses his analysis in statistical terms.

In the meantime, the clinician has developed insight from his empirical studies, which are not related to numbers. His contacts with his subject enable him to scan and pattern his clinical findings and to think of them in the form of descriptive statements. His task now is to reconcile the statistical findings with the empirically derived patterns. This often requires a choice of statistical results depending on the suitability of their fineness or coarseness.[13] In sum, the processes included in adequate research designs include observations, descriptions, ratings, coding and statistical methods.

Finally, the investigator reaches the stage of formulating his tentative explanations or conclusions based on the degrees of significance derived from the combined observational and statistical data. Significance may be sharply clear, or may only indicate trends. The investigator's proof, however, does not lie within his closed design. The validity of the results (qualitative or quantitative) depends on a confluence or correlation with other findings outside his own system indicating a sound relationship with data from other approaches and disciplines, using independent measures of the same thing. Nevertheless, to quote Harry Stack Sullivan,[14] "The principal increments in our understanding of mental disorder must for some considerable time come from the scientific acumen of clinical psychiatrists."

Checklist of Questions to Be Asked about a Research Program*

1. What is the problem?
   a. Is it clearly stated?
   b. Is it focused enough to facilitate efficient work (i.e., are hypotheses directly testable)?
2. What are the underlying objectives?
   a. Is the problem clearly related to the objectives?
3. What is the significance of the proposed research?
   a. How does it tie in with theory?
   b. What are its implications for application?
4. Has the relevant literature been adequately surveyed?
   a. Is the research adequately related to other people's work on the same or similar topics?
5. Are the concepts and variables adequately defined (theoretically and operationally)?
6. Is the design adequate?
   a. Does it meet formal standards for consistency, power, and efficiency?

*From R. R. Holt's chapter: "Experimental Methods in Clinical Psychology" in *Handbook of Clinical Psychology* edited by B. Wolman. Used with permission of McGraw-Hill Book Co., New York, N.Y., 1970 and the author.

    b. Is it appropriate to the problem and the objectives?

    c. Will negative results be meaningful?

    d. Are possibly misleading and confounding variables controlled?

    e. How are the independent and dependent variables measured or specified?

7. What instruments or techniques will be used to gather data?

    a. Are the reliabilities and validities of these techniques well established?

8. Is the sampling of subjects adequately planned for?

    a. Is the population (to which generalizations are to be aimed) specified?

    b. Is there a specific and acceptable method of drawing a sample from this population?

9. Is the sampling of objects (or situations) adequately planned for?

    a. To what population of objects (situations) will generalizations be aimed?

    b. Is there a specific and acceptable method of drawing a sample from this population?

10 What is the setting in which data will be gathered?

    a. Is it feasible and practical to carry out the research plan in this setting?

    b. Is the cooperation of the necessary persons obtainable?

11. How are the data to be analyzed?

    a. What techniques of "data reduction" are contemplated?

    b. Are methods specified for analyzing data qualitatively?

    c. Are methods specified for analyzing data quantitatively?

12. In the light of available resources, how feasible is the design?

    a. What compromises must be made in translating an idealized research design into a practical research design?

    b. What limitations or generalizations will result?

    c. What will be needed in terms of time, money, personnel, and facilities?

REFERENCES

1. Millon, T. *Theories of psychopathology and personality.* (2nd ed.) Philadelphia: W. B. Saunders, 1973.
2. Millon, T., & Diesenhaus, H. I. *Research methods in psychopathology.* New York: John Wiley, 1972.
3. Chassan, J. B. *Research design in clinical psychology and psychiatry.* New York: Appleton-Century-Crofts, 1967.
4. Sahakian, W. S. *Psychopathology today.* Itasca, Ill.: F. E. Peacock, 1970.
5. Offer, D., & Freedman, D. X. (Eds.) *Modern psychiatry and clinical research.* New York: Basic Books, 1972.
6. Anthony, E. J. Research as an academic function of child psychiatry. *Arch. Gen. Psych.,* 1969, **21**, 385–391.
7. Kaplan, A. *The conduct of inquiry.* San Francisco: Chandler, 1964.
8. Sargent, H. D. Intrapsychic change: methodological problems in psychotherapy research. *Psychiatry,* 1961, **24**, 93–109.
9. Mora, G., & Brand, J. L. (Eds.) *Psychiatry and its history.* Springfield, Ill.: Charles C. Thomas, 1970.
10. Hamburg, D. A., Sabshin, M. S., Board, F. A., Grinker, R. R., Sr., Korchin, S. J., Basowitz, H., Heath, H., & Persky, H. Classification and rating of emotional experiences. *Arch. Neurol. and Psych.,* 1958, **79**, 415–426.
11. Bruner, J., & Tagiuri, R. The perception of people. In G. Lindzey (Ed.), *Handbook of social psychology.* Vol. II, p. 634. Cambridge, Mass.: Addison-Wesley, 1954.

12. Heynes, R., & Lippitt, R. Systematic observational techniques. In G. Lindzey (Ed.), *Handbook of social psychology*, Vol. I, p. 370. Cambridge, Mass.: Addison-Wesley, 1954.
13. Grinker, R. R., Sr., Werble, B., & Drye, R. A. *The borderline syndrome.* New York: Basic Books, 1968.
14. Sullivan, H. S. The common field of research and clinical psychiatry. *Psychiatric Quarterly*, 1927, 1, 276–291.

VII

Normality

Comparison groups and normal controls are an essential part of most clinical research. For many researchers, however, locating normal subjects for control groups is a difficult task requiring time-consuming, careful screening of each subject. So many so-called normal or healthy persons who volunteer for a fee turn out to have serious elements of psychopathology. This seems to be especially true among contemporary college students.

"Normality" or "health" are two heavily value-laden terms, and they may be defined in various ways depending on the perspective of the investigator. To define mental health requires knowledge of the culturally embraced values held by subject-patient and observer-investigator. Subjects comprising a mentally healthy group do not show absolute mental health. It is far more appropriate to analyze the reciprocal and sequential relations among multiple variables to obtain typologies with probabilistic boundaries.

Yet until recently psychiatrists who were concerned primarily with psychopathology had implicitly assigned the field of "normality" to clinical psychology. In fact, when lay people became curious about the difference between clinical psychology and clinical psychiatry, they were usually told that the former deals with normal and the latter with pathological psychic states. Now, however, both fields are focusing on psychopathology.

In 1962, Grinker et al. [1,2] published two papers dealing with a normal, healthy population of young males who were attending a local college. Using a few of the young men, whom we had carefully screened, for normal controls in stress experiments, we found, to our astonishment, that the whole student body was as devoid of psychopathology as any group the authors had ever seen. The authors therefore studied them intensively by means of interviews, questionnaires and teachers' reports.

There was a general sense of stability occasioned by a good fit between the precollege life and goals and the environment of the college (George Williams); although there were, however, many individual differences and group differentiations into groups of very well-, fairly well- and marginally well-adjusted students. When special students attended classes at the nearby University of Chicago they were called "upright young men" and corresponded to Friedenberg's and Roth's "muscular Christians."[3] On the other hand, they were also similar to Silber et al.'s[4] "competent adolescents."

For over a decade we "forgot" our investigation on mentally healthy young males. The term "homoclites," which was invented to avoid the value judgments of the words "normality" or "health," was never picked up by anyone else and not used in any subsequent publication. In the meantime, we had finished programs of research on depressions and borderlines and then, 14 years later, we were confronted with the serious problem of obtaining normal controls for our research program on schizophrenia. Where could we find them?

We were studying young first-break hospitalized schizophrenics and had sufficient hospitalized nonschizophrenic controls. Suddenly we remembered the homoclites of 14 years ago, who at that time were about the same age as the current patients under study. We circulated a questionnaire to the 1959 subjects identical to the follow-up document filled out yearly by our research patients. Because we had deleted many last names of the homoclites from the original questionnaires, only 37 were matched with the original questionnaires. We then analyzed the unmatched ones in the same manner and achieved the same results thus giving us a total of 134 controls.[5]

Comparing the 1959 (published in 1962) with the 1973 data showed that four items indicated increased ego functioning and maturity, and seven comparisons showed no significant differences. In other words, the subjects either sustained their good health into the third decade of their adulthood or were improved. As a result, we have a normal control group of 134 males available for a variety of clinical investigations.

In the meantime psychiatric interest in normality became greatly stimulated and a number of studies were published. In our Institute, Offer and Sabshin[6] reviewed the literature and considered normality from the following four perspectives: 1) health; 2) utopia; 3) average; and 4) transactional (in relation to others). Offer then studied a group of modal adolescents falling in the middle group of a variety of psychological scales that indicated high and low polarities. He started with students in the first year of two high schools and utilized interviews, psychological tests, questionnaires and information from their teachers and families. The subjects were followed through high school and college and many are still being seen in postcollege, postwar and work situations. The data have indicated a high predictive value for future stability.[7]

There are many subsidiary conclusions from this research which indicate that normality is a pluralistic term dependent on combinations of varieties of culture, social expectations, value systems, professional biases, individual differences and political climates. Offer now possesses a normal control group for his current study of adolescent delinquents. Offer's major findings have been that his group experienced a relatively long period of adolescence. They proceeded through it slowly, mastering its various tasks gradually. As a result, they evidenced comparatively little turmoil. In other words, gradualism, as contrasted to volcanic eruptions, best typifies the developmental psychology of the normal adolescent sample.

Interviews, observations, questionnaires and psychological tests are standard methods for long-term research on normality and psychopathology, with one important addition. This is the "follow-up," which includes a highly technical and varied series of tactics requiring more than telephone calls or written inquiries. They require much time and patience. Without the necessary patience and skills Garber[8] could not have determined the long-term effect of hospitalizing adolescents and Werble[9] could not have proven that the "borderline syndrome" was not a phase of schizophrenia.

The health-illness systems cannot be separated to define health and illness each in absolute terms. Health is dependent on factors such as age, culture and social attitudes, internal compensations, defenses, coping, etc. In general, health is maintained when strains affecting one part of the biopsychological system are compensated for or counteracted by other parts. Even a new relationship between or disequilibrium of the parts caused by stress may ultimately develop into an adequate adaptation.

In general, the health-illness system involving body and mind extends from the genetic to the socio-cultural, and encompasses development and decline. This includes birth, infancy, childhood, adolescence, young adulthood, maturity, aging, dying and death. Each phase has its characteristic internal processes, its specific stresses and capacities for defense, coping and reconstitution. Each and the whole have their interfaces with specific socio-cultural environments, their ecological systems. This concept transcends disciplinary lines; it combines knowledge of laboratory procedures, life in pairs, families, groups and the larger society. It is concerned with phases of stability, stress-responses and despair.

Stages in the lifecycle considered as a system may be viewed in several ways. For example, from one point of view we may see the subsystem of ontogeny as including genetics (bioamines), family (communications) and experience (trauma), all being parts of ontogeny and all leading to health or illness and degrees of susceptibility to the latter and coping devices for the former.

Each phase has its genetic, environmental and experimental components, and to a point not yet understood, spontaneous movement and shifts due to intervention may occur. Corresponding to general systems theory, the principle of isomorphism of each level may be assumed. It is important for research and for the practical goals of therapy to incorporate phases of the individual lifecycle into our educational processes in universities and medical schools.[10]

It seems evident that social life structures opportunities for individual instinctual gratification, but it also frustrates by demanding many renunciations. The concept of balance between these polarities characterizes unitary thinking, although the empirical phenomena indicate that one or the other polarity dominated at various times in the history of each society. Society provides ego-ideals, ideologies and social roles for personality development, but the social structure is developed and is maintained by a variety of personality conglomerates.

It then may be assumed that, out of this matrix, factors promoting types of health and/or illness have great significance no matter how strong biogenetic defects may be.

Psychiatric problems arise out of a social matrix and in turn alter that matrix with the same reciprocity that articulates personality with society.

The relevance of social psychiatry in the development and persistence of deviant feeling, thinking and behavior is what concerns us. Extravagant claims have been made for community psychiatry without sound processes of evaluation, except in rare instances. Kellam and Branch[11] indicate that, currently, community psychiatry is a nonsystem in an experimental area where mental health is poorly defined except as internal wellbeing and appropriate adaptation.

If we knew the precise whats and hows of the influence deriving from the social matrix, however, it might be possible intentionally to prevent or even change those social and cultural factors that most significantly facilitate psychiatric problems and thus become a part of a system of health services and primary prevention. From a practical standpoint, the operations of so-called community psychiatry should be based on the characteristics of multiple subsystems within a community mental health center and on the transactions among various systems within special communities such as social agencies, police, courts, schools, churches, etc.

Experiences with "men under stress" and the results of other researchers indicated that emotional specificity in the production of psychosomatic disturbances is rare. Indeed, after much time, energy and work, we began to understand that a variety of stress stimuli could produce the same specific responses in each individual. The theory of *response specificity* was thus developed and perforce had to include the wide number of subsystems that preceded and contributed to classes of responses including experience, coping mechanisms and personality characteristics.

REFERENCES

1. Grinker, R. R., Sr., Grinker, R. R., Jr., & Timberlake, J. A study of mentally healthy young males (homoclites). *Arch. Gen. Psych.*, 1962, **6**, 405–453.
2. Grinker, R. R., Sr. A dynamic story of the homoclite. In J. Masserman(Ed.), *Science and psychoanalysis.* Vol. 6, pp. 115–134. New York: Grune & Stratton, 1962.
3. Friedenberg, E. Z., & Roth, J. A. *Self-perception in the university.* Chicago: University of Chicago Press, 1954.
4. Silber, E., Hamburg, D. A., Coelho, G. W., Murphy, E. B., Rosenberg, M., & Pearlin, I. Adaptive behavior in competent adolescents: coping and anticipation of college. *Arch. Gen. Psych.*, 1961, **5**, 517.
5. Grinker, R. R. Sr, & Werble, B. Mentally healthy young males (homoclites) 14 years later. *Arch. Gen. Psych.* 1974, **30,** 701–704.
6. Offer, D., & Sabshin, M. *Normality: theoretical and clinical concepts of mental health.* New York: Basic Books, 1966.
7. Offer, D. *The psychological world of the teen-ager.* New York: Basic Books, 1969.
8. Garber, B. *Follow-up study of hospitalized adolescents.* New York: Brunner/Mazel, 1972.
9. Werble, B. Second follow-up study of borderline patients. *Arch. Gen. Psych.*, 1970, **23**, 3–8.
10. Grinker, R. R., Sr. Biochemical education as a system. *Arch. Gen. Psych.*, 1971, **24,** 290–298.
11. Kellam, S. G., & Branch, J. D. Strategies in urban community mental health. In S. Golann, & C. Eisdorfer (Eds.), *Handbook of community psychology.* New York: Appleton-Century-Croft, 1971. 1971.

VIII

Biological Research

There seem to be no limits to the extent of biological research, or the extent to which it may become significant for psychiatry. Support for such investigations must not be based on the need to demonstrate so-called "relevance to the human condition." Even futurology, a new discipline that examines what the future may hold, cannot predict which laboratory, test or field observations may hold the key that will unlock the mysteries of human psychoses. The usual generalization of the futurologists is in essence: "More of the same and better than." Irrelevance is a contemporary judgment that may be correct or incorrect, stimulating or depressing for future activities.

According to Rainer,[1] genetics and psychiatry followed separate paths until the 1930's. At that time Nissl and Alzheimer described specific acute and chronic ganglion cell changes in the cerebral cortex. But, unfortunately, not one of these specific changes held up with subsequent research. Also, the notion that schizophrenics were congenitally deficient in specific areas such as the third layer of the cerebral cortex could never be confirmed. As a result of these failures, attention has been directed to neurochemical alterations of various types and locations, stimulated by the discovery of psychotropic drugs.

The nature-nurture dichotomy separated the biological and the psychological disciplines, and to some extent it still does, especially since many American psychoanalysts focus exclusively on psychogenesis—this despite the fact that Freud[2] himself wrote about the neuroses, "... They are severe, constitutionally fixed illnesses, which rarely restrict themselves to only a few attacks, but persist as a rule over long periods or throughout life." He further stated that we have neglected the constitutional factor in our therapeutic practice, and in any case we can do nothing about it; but in theory we ought to bear it in mind.

There are, however, indications that biological factors are increasingly being considered in the formulations of etiology of mental disturbances, and we are concerned with how genetics and environmentally induced experiences are interlocked. Rainer[1] states, "More than a static combination of two factors added together, the interaction is a continuous process with mutual feedback, and spiral development through a series of critical stages."

Are there neuropathological or neurophysiological alterations in the psychoses such as those Meltzer and Crayton[3] have shown to occur in the neuromuscular synapses, or do the psychoses involve damage to parts of the central nervous system preceded or followed by serious dysfunction? Or is the primary process one of disturbed central physiology? This is our modern neuropathology, which supercedes the morphological pathology that developed at Kraepelin's suggestion during the time of his early classifications. Each discipline among the biological sciences has a tremendous body of literature that cannot be currently evaluated. Later, in greater detail, we shall bring together the research that applies especially to schizophrenia.

A comparison between monozygotic and dizygotic twins reared by one or both parents with psychopathology raises many questions. Individual intrauterine trauma or circulatory disturbance, premature birth, tamponage on the head of the first twin through the birth canal, identical environments may result in effects not due to genetic identity. It may sometimes be difficult to determine mono- or dizygosity, especially since we have no certain method by which to determine gene structure or position. Thus, for twin studies, problems of sampling and lack of certainty of diagnosis are serious complications, so that conclusions regarding the variance contributed by heredity are widely different in different reports. The original statistics published by Kallman[4] on concordance rate of monozygotic twins for schizophrenia now seem too high.

Twin studies are also complicated by so-called "soft" signs of brain damage at birth or shortly after which are difficult to observe and quantify. Furthermore, these "soft" signs may be completely hidden by compensations and adjustments and not evident even by careful neurological examinations in later life.[5]

Twins are apt to be treated alike, so that the similar psychological influences may have more to do with concordance in monozygotic twins than the genetic factor.[6] The separation of twins by the adoption of one into a healthy family has been studied. Despite this salutary influence, the "experimental" group of children of schizophrenics had a significantly higher percentage of schizophrenia than did the normal controls (no schizophrenic parent). The index twin, whether at home or adopted, had a higher excretion level of catecholamines.[7]

Schildkraut and Kety[8] although showing that norepinephrine has an effect on emotions—decreasing them in depressions and increasing them in mania—state that this does not indicate a genetic or constitutional predomination; it may instead be due to early environmental factors. Wolpert[9] calls the manic-depressions, based on excess or inhibition of discharge of norepinephrine, an "actual neurosis" with symptoms secondarily invested with psychological meaning. Additional biological evidences are abnormal noctural EEG's, differences in sleep cycle and quality of dreams; failure of psychotherapy and success with lithium maintenance.[10] At any rate, we know that depressed patients show marked anxiety and elevation of 17 hydrocorticosteroids as they come out of their depressions, at which time they are most prone to suicide. A new method of research is oriented toward having healthy subjects "simulate" various moods to determine whether their biochemical processes change to the biochemistry that is found in the actual disease.

Winokur et al.[11] have indicated that manic-depressive patients have an earlier age of onset than do depressive patients, and that they also have an increased number of episodes of illness. Manic patients are more likely to have familial or parental affective disorder than are depressive patients. Winokur states:

In the families of bipolar (manic-depressive) patients, about a third of the affectively ill family members will have a mania, whereas about two-thirds of the family members will have had only depression. In the families of depressive patients there will be none or few manic family members. Consequently, manic-depressive disease can manifest itself as either a mania or a depression or both. Depressive disease manifests itself only by one or more depressions.

Other kinds of genetic studies have been done. In manic-depressive disease, several studies have shown that more women than men are ill. This suggests that X-linkage is involved. Two studies now have indicated that X-linkage is indeed involved in manic-depressive disease. Manic-depressive disease appears to be linked specifically to the loci for color blindness and the Xg-a blood group. Both of these markers are on the short end of the X-chromosome. Other clinical features have been found. There seems to be an increased prevalence of post partum episodes in manic depressives when compared to depressive disease patients.

As regards biological differences, studies indicate a decreased threshold to visual stimuli in bipolar as compared to unipolar patients. Bipolars have an augmenting pattern and unipolars a reducing pattern of the average cortical evoked response. Urinary excretion of 17-hydroxycorticosteroids may be reduced in a group of depressed bipolars as compared to depressed unipolars. The administration of L-dopa has been associated with mild hypomania or improvement in depression in bipolar patients. Unipolars have no antidepressant response to L-dopa. Thus there are indications of biological differences in the two clinical groups of affective disorders.

In summary, it would appear that using a genetic methodology, two types of affective disorders have been isolated by Winokur—*Manic*-depressive disease and *depressive* disease. Clinical and biological differences also seem to separate these two groups. It is entirely likely that in the course of time there will be differential responses to treatment in these groups.

Kety indicates that there is an increased awareness of the complexity of biochemical mechanisms in mental diseases. He too considers, for example, schizophrenia as a polygenetic inadequacy interacting with particular life situations. Among the biochemical substances accused of playing a role in the development of psychoses are proteins, amino acids and amines, transmethylization abnormalities, indole amines and norepinephrine. One of the huge problems in attributing the position of genetic and biochemical defects in the etiology of disease is the poor sampling of index cases and the limited follow-up. Thus the manifestations of these diseases are both genetic and psychological. The depressions may be a derivative of the "sulk-prone" child, or may involve the mother changing from a giving person to an expecting person.

So far as the EEG is concerned, research on the average evoked response has as yet revealed no differences between schizophrenia and other diseases. Giannitrapani and Kayton[12] used a digital spectrum analysis of hospitalized adolescent or young schizophrenics in remission from an acute psychotic episode. With this complicated method and analysis they found significant differences in the location of the bands of dominant alpha frequency.

The circulating and excreted proteins, vitamins and enzymes have been studied by many investigators with contradictory results. As Mandell[13] states:

> We have turned from the search for psychotoxins to a focus on the pathophysiology of adaptational processes. There appears to be little question that an important portion of neurochemical research will be focused on regulation and adaptation in the years to come.

Psychopharmacology, in its development of tranquilizers against anxiety, anti-depressive drugs, lithium against manias and phenothiazines against the disorganization of schizophrenics, has been extremely valuable for therapy. In fact, there is considerable evidence from double blind studies, placebo controls in randomized crossover studies and control of potency, that these drugs are more effective than any form of psychotherapy—although the most effective treatment may be drugs and psychotherapy in combination. The investigations of the psychotropic drugs have enormously stimulated the field of neurochemistry. The pertinent question is, where do these drugs act? Do they affect certain types of fibers or cells, or do they act on specific structures of the central nervous system such as the hypothalamus[14] or the limbic lobe? These are important questions that have stimulated much research.

Other biological studies have been published from time to time, but never verified. Williams[15] relates constitution to specific personalities. His formula is: genes give rise to enzymes that create various nutritional needs such as those that give rise to alcoholism. Sheldon[16] correlates body build, derived from an intricate series of measurements with personality, temperament, etc. Kurt Goldstein[17] working with brain-damaged persons, correlates their catastrophic reactions, anxiety and concrete thinking with similar findings in schizophrenics.

Ashby[18] dichotomizes activities of the nervous system into reflex behavior and learned behavior not inborn and not specified by the gene pattern. He asks why learned behavior is usually a change toward better adaptation. He defines environment as those variables whose changes affect the organism, and those variables which are changed by the organism's behavior. Psychiatrists immersed in psychopathology would not accept the concept of "usually changed for the better." Concerning learned behavior, the ethologists[19] have studied early imprinting on experimental animals. The field is highly controversial and application to man has not yet been verified.

In conclusion, we have indicated some aspects of biological research in general, but certainly not all, since there are many subdisciplines and many methods in the field, all or any of which may contribute to our future understanding of mental illness. However, as Vale[20] states, "The major question is how does the genotype or the resulting biochemical processes combine with the environment to produce the behavioral process?" We shall discuss this further in Chapter XIII.

REFERENCES

1. Rainer, J. D. Genetics and psychiatry. In A. Friedman & H. Kaplan (Eds.), *Comprehensive psychiatry*. New York: Williams & Wilkins, 1973.

2. Freud, S. New introductory lectures on psychoanalysis. In J. Strachey (Ed. and translator) *Standard Edition.* Vol. 22. London: Hogarth Press, 1964.
3. Meltzer, H., & Crayton, J. Muscle abnormality in psychotic patients. Serum CPK activity, fiber abnormalities and branching and sprouting of subterminal nerves. *(in press)*
4. Kallmann, F. *Heredity in health and mental disorder.* New York: W. W. Norton, 1953.
5. Pasamanick, B., & Knobloch, H. Retrospective studies on the epidemiology of reproductive causality: old and new. *Merril-Palmer Quart. of Behavior and Development,* 1966, **1**, 7–26.
6. Kringlen, E. Schizophrenia in twins. *Psychiatry,* 1966, **29**, 172–184.
7. Rosenthal, D. Problems of sampling and diagnosis in the major twin studies of schizophrenia. *Journal of Psychiatric Research,* 1961, **1**, 116–134.
8. Schildkraut, J. J., & Kety, S. S. Biogenetic amines and emotion. *Science,* 1956, **156**, 21–30.
9. Wolpert, E. A. Manic depressive illness as an "actual" neurosis. *(in press)*
10. Wolpert, E. A. Psychophysiological parallelism in the dream. In L. E. Abt, & B. F. Riess (Eds.), *Progress in Clinical Psychology.* Vol. VIII. *Dreams and Dreaming.* New York: Grune & Stratton, 1968.
11. Winokur G., Clayton, P. J., & Reich, T. *Manic depressive illness.* St. Louis: C. V. Mosby, 1969.
12. Giannitrapani, D. & Kayton, L. Schizophrenic and EEG spectrum analysis. *E. E. G. and Clinical Neurophysiology.* 1974, **36**, 377–386.
13. Mandell, A. J., Segal, D. S., Kuczenski, R. T., & Knapp. S. The search for the schizococcus. In R. Cancro (Ed.), *Annual Review of the Schizophrenic Syndrome.* Vol. 3. New York: Brunner/Mazel, 1973.
14. Grinker, R. R., Sr. Electroencephographic studies of corticohypothalamic relations in schizophrenia. *American Journal of Psychiatry,* 1941, **98**, 37.
15. Williams, R. J. *Biochemical individuality.* New York: John Wiley, 1953.

16. Sheldon, W. H. Constitutional psychiatry. In T. Millon (Ed.), *Theories of psychopathology and personality.* (2nd ed.) Philadelphia: W. B. Saunders, 1973.
17. Goldstein, K. *The organism: a holistic approach to biology.* New York: American Book Co., 1939.
18. Ashby, W. R. *Design for a brain.* New York: John Wiley, 1965.
19. Tinbergen, N. *The study of instinct.* New York: Oxford University Press, 1951.
20. Vale, J. R. Role of behavior genetics in psychology. *American Psychologist,* 1973, **28,** 871–882.

IX

Early Experiences, Psychoanalysis and Intrapsychic Processes

Although we know that the biology and constitution of the child at birth determine its predisposition or lack of it for future mental illness or "normality," the child's early experiences constitute the stimuli that activate the process. Unfortunately, the retrospective information obtained from the adolescent or young adult is not accurate and the parents' accounts of early experience are frequently distorted, forgotten or altered in self protection.

Shakow[1] suggests that, for this period, direct observation of child development and parenting be conducted in the home by means of video-tape recording, especially during the intense phase of psychomotor and language development that occurs in the second year of life, also a time when mother's actions are important models. Shakow suggests that instead of Freud's emphasis on trauma and isolated events, William James's[2] ideas on the incidental, minimal reiterated small accretions of competence be observed and recorded. He does acknowledge that this constitutes an invasion of privacy and facilitates the projection of the observer's bias. Shakow suggests greater emphasis on individ. uality than on the nomothetic, more importance to extremes than the averages of behavior and more attention to invulnerability than to damage.

It seems clear that child observations should become a more significant type of research in the field of child development. Piaget[3] has accomplished a great deal by studying cognitive development but few other investigators are interested or competent to study psychomotor and affective development. An obvious exception is Spitz's[4] study of infants in foundling homes who were not held, cuddled or soothed by substitute mothers, resulting in marasmus and death of the child. Or Bowlby's[5] studies of infants separated from their mothers or Harlow's[6] experiments on monkeys removed from their mothers but maintained in good nutrition, with devastating results in later life.

In this period we do have to take into account the early infection, metabolic disturbances,[7] trauma, rejecting and hostile mothers. Many of these experiences are difficult to pinpoint in retrospect. Furthermore, child psychiatrists are less interested in well-babies than in psychopathology, but clinical psychologists seem to fill in the gap in this field. Included in these early experiences are the studies of pathological families as units predisposing to the development of schizophrenia. These findings will be described in a subsequent chapter.

The question of whether psychoanalysis can revive, within the transference neurosis, new editions of old infantile and childhood experiences and their reactive feelings, will now be considered. Unfortunately, these interpretations are colored by considerable bias, and explanations may have little to do with causes. Psychoanalysis is a discipline that has contributed more to clinical psychiatry then any other. Yet since Freud's early theoretical formulation, psychoanalytic theory has been a mixture of old, abandoned or modified concepts with newer accretions. It is not a unified theory, but is composed of often unrelated part-theories. Psychoanalysis is not a single package, which makes it difficult to pinpoint testable hypotheses.[8]

Indeed, psychoanalysts have been hostile to any scientific studies of what they call "Our Science," as if scientific inquiry would vitiate the intuition of the practitioner. Glover[9] states harshly that, "Psychoanalysts maintain an unrestricted license to interpret which results in a degree of fabrication that violates their conclusions." The organizational die-hards attempt to exclude others who would attempt to effect change and perhaps even progress.

There seem to be three periods in Freud's own theoretical development. The first period includes concepts of a dynamic unconscious, motivation, genetic infantile experiences and primary and secondary process thinking. The second period includes the theory of anxiety, defense mechanisms and the creation of a metapsychology serving as an umbrella for dynamic, psychogenic, structural, economic and adaptive subtheories. At this time, about 1920, Freud ceased publishing *clinical* data.[10] The third period, which extends to the present and has been greatly amplified by Hartman,[11] is called the era of ego psychology.

Percival Bailey[12] severely criticized psychoanalysis as a closed system but Grinker[13] showed how the field was first an open system, closing abruptly with the development of the dual instinct theory (never fully accepted) and opened again with the development of the tripartite structural theory and the principle of adaptation. A brilliant parody on this was written by John Millet.[14] On the other hand, Gitelson[15] states, "None of us can say that we are not disillusioned. Unfortunately many have also been bitterly disappointed. The difference is between insight and transference reaction." Those who criticize have transference reactions, and then he says, "Paradoxically, but not incomprehensible to psychoanalysts, the child, psychiatry, has turned against the father while accepting its birthright."

One of the most significant barriers against bringing psychoanalytic theory and research in line with other sciences is its insistence on libido or psychic energy. But instinctual processes may be considered as communication systems. The distortions in development of instinctual processes, rather than libidinal conflicts, are better determinants of different healthy and pathological forms of communications. Quantities may be expressed in terms of too much or too little, too early or too late, or of distortions. Psychic energy, a reductionistic term based on nineteenth-century physics, prevents bridges with other sciences. It is bad biology and should be abandoned for the sake of a proper biological psychiatry.

> Modern psychoanalysis requires field theory to include the transactions among multiple functions—genic, developmental, organ activities, hormones, nervous system, mental structures, social, cultural and physical environment—and to account for degrees of health and illness. One system does not exclude the other and one alone cannot tell the whole story. How do we view the human being as a system in transaction instead of as a fractionated structure? We can view his genic system, his hormonal system, his nervous system, or his mental systems independently by means of special techniques as systems in their own right. Our modern task is to view these systems as parts of a larger whole by systematically studying the relationships among them. We do this by correlations of changes over specified time, changes in response to strains of development or to other stresses which disturb equilibrium.
>
> Operationally the whole human being and his many subsystems can fruitfully be viewed as a behaving organism utilizing thoughts, feelings, gestures, postures, and total movement in relation to a variety of others in his surrounding world. Behaviors of all kinds, not only verbal, communicate information re-

garding all component aspects of personality, drives, conflicts, defense, ideals, since the ego functions as the final common pathway—in and out—of personality traits and states. Behaviors reveal dilemmas, liabilities, assets, and compromises of the person in action. Therein lies the field for future study, awaiting appropriate scientific methods which are unbiased with regard to any specific theory.[16]

The psychoanalytic literature seems interminably involved with theory, repeating Freud's contributions and adding relatively little new. Basch,[17] however, has contributed new approaches in the last decade by considering syndromes as general systems dysfunctions and symbols as metaphors. But where is the research inspired by and derived from theory?

Sargent[18] introduced a research project which dealt with therapy in a problem-centered manner to determine how processes change and what factors change outcome. The results were assessed by using impressions judged by clinicians, calibrated by observations subject to methods for establishing reliability, validity and predictive accuracy.

On the same note of general systems theory, Gedo and Goldberg[19] have utilized a number of the component psychoanalytic theories, as they have been evolved by Freud, and created several models of the mind applied in a line of vertical maturation, facilitating a new taxonomy based on development, stages of regression, supraordinate controls and indicating forms of treatment for each stage.

This *assumes importance* for the behavioral scientist whose extrapsychoanalytic research may key into any point (a model or a stage of maturity) using his own concepts, hypotheses, tools, and criteria of validity. He then participates in a well-defined area, not in an amorphous jungle, and he can make systematic observations of specific phenomena. His position can be defined and what he observes can be focal. (Grinker[19])

Freud[20] contended that mental processes (probably meaning symbolic thinking) were unconscious and that perception of them by consciousness should be compared with the perception of the outside world through the sense organs. Psychoanalysis is a technique of introspection, and the environmental variables are represented by nonobjective memory-rests in the internal psychic life.

As Millon[21] points out, splinter groups detached themselves over time from the main body of psychoanalysis: the mysticism of Jung, Horney's sociocultural point of view, the Rankian birth-trauma, the philosophy of Erich Fromm and the interpersonal concepts of Sullivan. Most significant is Erikson's psychological stages of life-in-development such as basic trust *vs,* mistrust, autonomy *vs,* shame and doubt, initiative *vs,* guilt, industry *vs,* inferiority and identity *vs,* identity diffusion.[22]

In a recent publication of *Psychological Issues,* Mayman,[24] Spence and Gordon, Luborsky, Shevrin, Holzman and Meehl discuss psychoanalytic research. Clearly, railing against the absence of good research (the patient is not an unbiased collaborator) in the field cannot detract from the extensive and depth-like influence of psychoanalysis on all the behavioral sciences. Freud repeatedly wrote that his system had few *a priori* basic concepts and that it kept close to immediate observations using the psychoanalytic method. Yet, 1) it is used only for sick persons and 2) it is entirely private and not observable. Freud angrily rejected the use of experimental methods for purposes of validation (personal commication).

Let us now turn to what others have written about "dilution." Kubie, who is highly critical, states that "other sciences will clarify what is confused and muddy in psychoanalytic theory, concepts and terminology and will furnish material for critical self-examination." Sandford believes that "other methods besides the psychoanalytic one are useful for testing psychoanalytic hypotheses and that these hypotheses are no less psychoanalytic for being tested outside the consulting room." Stanton advocates using methods not characteristically psychoanalytic. Pumpian-Mindlin stated that psychoanalysis as a model is a closed system which blocks certain observations. Hartman admits that distortions of self-observation as well as of observations of others may occur. Bellak likewise critically states that psychoanalysts are applied scientists, professionals or therapists, and as such are sometimes ambivalent in their attitude toward theory, and are poorly trained in scientific methods, concept formation, or other rigors of thought taught to graduate students of science. As Bellak states, clinicians in general and psychoanalysts in particular are wary of the academic approach. (All the above are cited from discussions in Hook.)[25]

Colby[26] writes that psychoanalysis is a branch of science still trying to "develop scientific methods appropriate to its data and problems." It proposes a system of theory and observations about human behavior. The training of psychoanalysts has been limited for the most part to the transmission of this system without encouragement of original work. Low-level observational statements refer to what persons actually say or do in the psychoanalytic situation. Observations should be systematic, recorded and controlled. They may include the use of tape recorders and multiple observers. However, experimental observation remains an undeveloped aspect of psychoanalysis. Colby further states that theoretical biases have maintained the Freudian dual instinct theory using unrecorded observations, lack of quantification, lack of experimentation, lack of controls, lack of follow-up, lack of cooperative research, lack of predictive statements, lack of interpretive ruses and with obscurantist language.

Rapaport[28] states, despite the fact that Freud said that psychoanalytic theory can be validated only by the psychoanalytic method (and he says it has), that independent confirmation is needed by direct observation on infants and children. Psychoanalysis has no learning theory of its own. The field is beginning to extract valid contributions from theories of the neofreudian schools. These are statements from a leading psychoanalytic theoretician.

Finally, the editors of *Psychological Issues* (cf especially vol 4, No 1, "The Influence of Freud on American Psychology" by David Shakow and David Rapaport) agree that "relevant contributions can come from experimental studies as well as from genetic explorations of psychoanalytic therapy, and that investigations carried out without any concern for psychoanalysis may nevertheless contribute to the theory. . . ."

I take much pleasure in the fact that currently some psychoanalysts are developing the courage to question the fundamental concepts in the field. For example, Roy Schafer[29] writes of "the sorely needed updating of psychoanalytic language." He proposes, as does Ruesch, an action language. Emanuel Peterfreund[30] writes about "Information, Systems and Psychoanalysis." Among others I might mention Holzman,[23] Mayman,[24] Gedo and Goldberg[19] and the list is growing. Maybe, and hopefully, life is stirring in a scientifically almost moribund field which has contributed so much in the past to psychiatry and the humanities.

There are several disciplines with a wide variety of methods applicable to psychoanalytic research. For example, animal experimentation with motherless monkeys, observations on child development and behavior, biochemical variations during various stages of consciousness, EEG studies, etc. A good example is the finding that rejection arouses compensatory unconscious fantasies of being fed. But it is essential that the nonanalytic investigator know what portion of the conglomerate psychoanalytic theory he is using, never all of it. He often has to use tape recorders and auditory and visual observers of the psychoanalytic situation itself.

Holzman[23] points out the difficulties of psychoanalytic research. These include inadequate clinical training of investigators, poor scientific training of investigators, poor scientific training in psychoanalytic institutes and a narrow concept of research tasks. "What is needed is a sophisticated awareness of psychoanalytic ideas with investigatory skills." Eissler,[31] who has been a devout follower of Freud, states: "The psychoanalytic situation has already given forth everything it contains. It is depleted regarding research possibilities, at least as the possibility of new paradigms[26] is concerned." Kardiner, one of Freud's earliest American students, in a personal communication stated that psychoanalysis is dead unless it becomes an empirical discipline and he considers that its integrative processes require intense study of dreams.

Paul Meehl[27] summarizes the problem: "How do we get the advantages of having a skilled observer, who knows what to listen for and how to classify it, without having the methodological disadvantage that anyone who is skilled in this way has been theoretically brain-washed in the course of his training?" In Meehl's view, this is the methodological problem in psychoanalytic research.

Gill[32] has attempted to equate psychoanalytic structural theory with a theory of systems involving modes of function (process) and modes of organization (structure). Indeed, there are indications that other more scientific psychoanalysts have utilized some aspects of general systems theory in their writings. Among the most erudite is Frenkel-Brunswik,[33] who wrote about psychoanalysis and the unity of science. Colby[34] has done considerable research on psychoanalysis and information theory. Sullivan[35] groped in this direction when he considered schizophrenia as a human process. Pumpian-Mindlin[36] attempted to relate psychoanalysis with biological and social sciences and Beres[37] considered an ego system of structure-function in psychoanalysis. Finally, Anna Freud[38] defined openness and multifactorial process in growth and development, in health and illness, and in therapeutic success and failure as hypotheses essential for testing of psychoanalytic theory by a variety of methods. Nevertheless, psychoanalysts have tried to force biology, physiology and evolutionary time into a world the center of which is the mind of man. As we have read many times, beginning with Sherrington,[39] "psychic energy" has no relation to physical energy.

REFERENCES

1. Shakow, D. Some thoughts about schizophrenia research in the context of high risk studies. *Psychiatry,* 1973, **36,** 353–366.
2. James, W. *The principles of psychology.* (Originally published 1890.) New York: Henry Holt & Co., 1950.
3. Piaget, J. *Origins of intelligence in children.* New York: International Universities Press, 1951.
4. Spitz, R. A. Relevancy of direct infant observations. *Psychoanal. Study of the Child,* 1950, **5,,** 66–75.
5. Bowlby, J. The nature of the child's tie to his mother. *Int. Journ. Psychoanal.* 1958, **39,** 350–373.
6. Harlow, H., & Harlow, M. K. Learning to love. *American Scientist,* 1966, **5,** 244–272.
7. Grinker, R. R., Sr. The effect of infantile disease on ego patterns. *Amer. Journ. of Psychiatry,* 1953, **110,** 290–295.
8. Madison, P. *Freud's concept of repression and defense.* Minneapolis: University of Minnesota Press, 1961.
9. Glover, E. *On the early development of the mind.* London: Harcourt, Brace, 1933.
10. Gedo, J. E., Sabshin, M., Sadow, L., & Schlessinger, N. Studies on hysteria. *Journ. Amer. Psychoanalytic Assoc.,* 1964, **12,** 734–751.
11. Hartman, H. *Essays on ego psychology.* New York: International Universities Press, 1964. Also *Ego psychology and the problem of*

adaptation. Translated by D. Rapaport. New York: International Universities Press, 1953.

12. Bailey, P. The great psychiatric revolution. *Amer. Journ. Psych.*, 1956, **113,** 387. Also *Sigmund the unserene: tragedy in three acts.* Springfield, Ill.: C. C. Thomas, 1965.

13. Grinker, R. R., Sr. Conceptual progress in psychoanalysis. In J. Marmor (Ed.), *Modern psychoanalysis.* New York: Basic Books, 1968.

14. Millet, J. A. P. Psychoanalyticus Americanus—myth for reality. *Fortschritte der Psychoanalyse,* 1966, **2,** 54.

15. Gitelson, M. Communication from the president about neoanalytic movement. *Int. J. Psychoanal.,* 1962, **43,** 373.

16. Grinker, R. R., Sr. Identity or regression in American psychoanalysis. *Arch. Gen. Psych.,* 1965, **12,** 113–125.

17. Basch, M. Psychoanalysis and theory formulation. *Annual of psychoanalysis.* Vol I. New York: Quadrangle/New York Times Books, 1973.

18. Sargent, H. Intrapsychic change: methodological problems in psychotherapy research. *Psychiatry,* 1966, **24,** 93–109.

19. Gedo, J. E., & Goldberg, A. *Models of the mind: a psychoanalytic theory.* Chicago: University of Chicago Press, 1973.

20. Freud, S. New introductory lectures on psychoanalysis. In J. Strachey (Ed. and translator), *Standard Edition.* Vol. 22. London: Hogarth Press, 1964.

21. Millon, T. *Theories of psychopathology and personality.* (2nd ed.) Philadelphia: W. B. Saunders, 1973.

22. Erikson, E. (Ed.) Identity and the life cycle. *Psychological Issues,* Monograph 1, New York: International Universities Press, 1959.

23. Holzman, P. S. In M. Mayman (Ed.), Psychoanalytic research: three approaches to the study of subliminal processes. *Psychological Issues,* Monograph 30. New York: International Universities Press, 1973, p. 88.

24. Mayman, M. (Ed.) Psychoanalytic research: three approaches to the study of subliminal processes. *Psychological Issues,* Monograph 30. New York: International Universities Press, 1973.

25. Hook, S. (Ed.) *Psychoanalysis, scientific method and philosophy.* New York: Grove Press, 1960.

26. Colby, K. M. *Introduction to psychoanalytic research.* New York: Basic Books, 1960.
27. Meehl, P. E. In M. Mayman, *op. cit.,* p. 104.
28. Rapaport, D. Structure of psychoanalytic theory: systematizing attempt. In S. Koch (Ed.), *Psychology: a study of a science.* Vol. 3. New York: McGraw-Hill, 1963.
29. Schafer, R. The idea of resistance. *International Journal of Psychoanalysis,* 1973, **54,** 259–287.
30. Peterfreund, E. *Information, systems and psychoanalysis.* New York: International Universities Press, 1971.
31. Eissler, K. R. Irreverent remarks about the present and future of psychoanalysis. *Int. J. Psychoanal.,* 1969, **50,** 461–471.
32. Gill, M. Topography and systems in psychoanalytic theory. *Psychological Issues,* Monograph 10. New York: International Universities Press, 1963.
33. Frenkel-Brunswik, E. Psychoanalysis and the unity of science. *Proceedings of the American Academy of Arts and Sciences.* 1952.
34. Colby, K. M. Research in psychoanalytic information theory. *American Scientist,* 1961, **49,** 358–369.
35. Sullivan, H. S. *Schizophrenia as a human process.* New York: W. W. Norton, 1962.
36. Pumpian-Mindlin, E. The position of psychoanalysis in relation to the biological and social sciences. In E. Pumpian-Mindlin (Ed.), *Psychoanalysis as science.* Palo Alto: Stanford University Press, 1952.
37. Beres, D. Structure and function in psychoanalysis. *International Journal of Psychoanalysis,* 1965, **46,** 53–63.
38. Freud, A. *Normality and pathology in childhood.* New York: International Universities Press, 1965.
39. Sherrington, C. *Man on his nature.* Cambridge, Eng.: Cambridge University Press, 1940.

X

Social and Cultural
Techniques Applied to
Psychiatry

I have previously stated that health and illness develop from within the social and cultural milieu of the human child. A successful organismic-environmental relationship is conducive to the development of inner self-esteem and social competence; resulting behaviors affect both the individual and society.

Hamburg,[1] in a study of *behavioral genetics* using chimpanzees showed that the mother-infant relationship increasingly depends—to an extent increasing with time—on the reciprocal adaptation between this dyad and the whole group. The long period of immaturity and dependency is utilized for learning, as in the human, preparing the young for adult life—that which Hamburg calls "behavioral rehearsal." This involves play, exploratory behavior, observation, imitation and practice. All this could not be successful if it were not for the capacity of the whole group to protect the young. I quote Hamburg directly:

> To illustrate the way in which knowledge about primate behavior may be relevant to man, let us review

131

briefly what is known about the primate equivalent of
what is clearly a major current social problem for man,
namely destructive aggression. When are primates
likely to threaten and fight each other, or to threaten
and fight members of other species? The following is
a summary of situations likely to elicit such behavior
in chimpanzees.

When there is competition over food, especially if
highly desirable foods are spatially concentrated
or in short supply;

When an infant is being defended by its mother;

If a contest occurs over the dominance prerogatives
of two individuals of similar social rank;

As a redirection of aggression; for example, when a
low-ranking male has been attacked by a high-
ranking male, it often turns to attack an individual
subordinate to itself;

With failure of one animal to comply with a signal
given by the aggressor;

When a familiar animal appears strange or different;
for example, due to paralytic disease;

When changes in dominance status occur, over
time, especially among the adolescent and young
adult males;

When a female in estrus does not respond to an
adult male's courtship;

When relative strangers meet;

In the hunting and killing of small animals;

When a chimpanzee is suffering from a presumably
painful injury.

If one surveys the contexts listed above in which
aggressive behavior is most likely to occur in the natu-

ral habitat, much of the information can be condensed into two general categories: 1) defense; and 2) access to valued resources. Within each of these categories, a variety of animals or objects or activities may be involved. So behaving aggressively in contexts of defense and of access to valued resources may well have given selective advantage in the zoological sense to higher primates. In effect, such behavior, if adequately regulated, can be an enforcer of many adaptive requirements, such as those involving food, water, and protection from predators.

Although the study of primates closest to man in the evolutionary scale promises to add much to our knowledge of man's success or failure in coping, sociology (which includes anthropology and culture in our definition) has only begun its contribution. Parsons,[2] on the other hand, removes culture from action systems, although they interpenetrate. "The only real human 'specialization' is culture."

Parsons differentiated social systems from culture, defining the latter as a shared and transmitted set of meaning patterns in a society represented by symbols which are internalized in personalities and institutionalized in social systems. In behavior systems culture is analogous to the gene. . . . Culture has many different levels of generality and specificity, yet within each there is a normative element. A social system is organized about a common culture of its own; those who do not recognize these norms are outside a boundary. The unit of society is a human individual. It is a *role* in a particular behavioral system. Boundaries may be said to exist between differentiated social systems in a society, characterized by mobility and interpenetrability. Boundaries exist between social systems and personality systems which are not only interdependent but also interpenetrate. The role is the unit of social system but only part of the personality. (Grinker[3])

As John Spiegel[4] stated,

The link between psyche and group is established through group membership roles. Fathers and sons, leaders and followers, hosts and guests are names for members in formal and informal small groups, and they prescribe the kind of behavior expected from the role incumbent.

In Spiegel and Bell's[5] work on disturbed families, they found attempts on the part of the family (Irish and Italian) to engage in rapid social change into American middle-class patterns without understanding the values patterning the roles. Expectations gave rise to role conflicts.

During World War II, Grinker and Spiegel[6] were forced to deal with the environment as a source of stress-stimuli, especially in the psychiatric disturbances that were not specifically precipitated by combat experiences. We predicted in 1945 the social stressful conditions that did indeed play an important role in psychiatric problems of society 25 years later. By 1967 it could be stated with a degree of certainty that:

A living organism is not a self-acting system, and neither in growth and maintenance can it be torn from its environment with which it forms a so-called system; it is an open system with constant exchange with the physical and living world.[3]

The problem in the twentieth century is to bring the diversity of living systems now subserved by specific disciplines, each communicating with its own scientific jargon about a part of the whole, under the umbrella of a unified theory and related to each other through a bridging dynamic scientific language.[2]

Personality and social systems are in constant interaction.[7] The living organism's social relations are involved in complex organizations whose inner psychology and somatic functions make possible his variable activities. This requires a unitary approach placing physical, physiological and social events within one system of denotation. Communications systems should be defined as the setting or situation, the sender, his intent, the interpretation of the receiver, the agreement between sender and receiver, the media used and the metacommunication or instructions about the messages. All these factors are explicitly defined in Grinker, *et al.*[8]

According to Thompson,[9] a multidisciplinary viewpoint considers that a local community-in-environment is exclusively neither a physicochemical nor a societal system, but a structural-functional web-of-life and an integral part of a larger whole. Each local community is specialized to some degree, attempting to maintain its homeostasis when upset by active efforts toward change. Within this community web-of-life, the individual has the responsibility of coping.

Thompson enumerates six dimensions: the ecological, the somatic, the sociological, the symbolic, the psychic and the core values. Appropriate research methods are being developed for each dimension that are applicable to the behaviors characteristic of these dimensions. These behaviors include beliefs and values, tools, arts, crafts and literature. Culture may change under stress by means of symbolic adaptation. Thompson states:

> Healthy communities use their culture as a problem-solving medium, apply their traditional cultural patterns to new situations and change them realistically to resolve the changing problem situations appropriately.

Social psychiatry is the study of the etiology and dynamics of persons seen in their total environmental settings. It is etiological in aim if employing cultural anthropologists, sociologists, individual psychologists, biostatisticians and the insights of clinical psychiatrists. Levy and Rowitz[10] indicate four levels of research:

1. Any empirical phenomena
2. Any specific living empirical phenomena
3. Any specific empirical social phenomena
4. Any specific empirical phenomena applied to humans.

Transcultural psychiatry attempts to determine the influences on humans of similar and different cultures to determine what element of mental disorder is culture "fair" or culture "free."[11]

Many sociologists have approached the problems of determining society's influence on personality and psychological deviance by statistical means, in an effort to imitate the "hard" sciences; in this way, however, the core of the individual in the community web-of-life is lost. On the other hand, students such as Cottle[12] have worked with and in small groups observing, listening and noting what the individuals think, feel and do under various circumstances. Likewise, Minuchin[13] applies social methods in the study of the behavior of families with a psychosomatically ill child.

One of the first studies of epidemiology applied to mental diseases was made by Faris and Dunham[14] between 1922 and 1934 and published in 1959. It is usually referred to as the "Chicago area research," because it demarcated areas in that city with the highest rate of psychoses, especially schizophrenia. It demonstrated the demographic and social characteristics of areas where many cases were found, contrasting them with areas with few cases. The most frequent incidence of psychosis was found in Chicago's "skid-row" area, giving rise to the so-called "drift" hypothesis which indicated that those who suffer from serious mental disorders tend to seek the lowest social existence, living on occasional work, free food, "flop houses" and wine.

Hollingshead and Redlich[15] studied social class and mental disease in New Haven, Connecticut, and came to the conclusion that greater frequency of mental disorder occurs among the lower social classes. Here the question arises about the lack of education and the difficulty in communication. The social factors involved in psychosomatic diseases will be discussed in a later chapter.

Levy and Rowitz,[10] working in Illinois, knew that since the work of Dunham and Faris the mentally ill patients moved to other areas, so they studied the ecological characteristics of communities that produced differential rates. Their complicated statistical methods showed that the highest rates of schizophrenia occurred in disorganized communities in a great state of poverty. They subscribe to the hypothesis of social responses rather than social causation. Frequency was greater among men who were single, separated or divorced. The highest per capita rate of mental illness among blacks was in areas of low black population. The black subjects were more often diagnosed as schizophrenic, while the whites were more often alcoholic. These data suggest the "drift" hypothesis, in that individuals were extruded from cohesive social structures. The criticism of this work, as well as other epidemiological studies, is its dependence on hospital admission diagnoses and the inadequate American Psychiatric Association nosological classification.

Cooper and Morgan's[16] recent monograph is the most complete one on the subject at this time. They demonstrate a correlation between a particular poverty-stricken lifestyle and a prevalence of mental illness in general, but not specifically with schizophrenia or manic-depressive psychoses. Their data identify each person, using techniques of sociology, psychology, public health, genetics and biostatistics—because epidemiology is a "collective science." It is a basic public health science study of distribution of disease in time and space, and of the factors that influence this distribution. Unfortunately, clinical diagnoses are so insecure that the authors hope that definitive biological markers will be found.

Epidemiological methods utilize surveys of prevalence at a point of time, follow-up of high risk patients and rates of new cases using modern sampling techniques and case registries. Precise definition for positive case identification depends on screening procedures, case-finding, rating scales, interviews and questionnaires. The results could be useful in planning, evaluation, prevention, prognosis and prediction of risk. Thus, epidemiology is an essential part of psychiatry as a system.

Clausen writes:[17]

> I would emphasize again the importance of the models of personality development and of psychopathology underlying ecological and epidemiological studies of mental illness. We have a great deal of evidence that different aspects of socio-cultural environment are implicated in the etiology of different types of psychopathological illness and in subsequent responses to the manifestations of such illness. As we learn to make more meaningful classifications of illness, whether we are dealing with disease entities or reaction tendencies, it will be possible to delineate more clearly the social ecology of particular types of mental illness. Ecological and epidemiological studies can themselves contribute to improvements in classification insofar as they reveal the social processes which influence recognition of constellations of cases. If this assessment is correct, we face a long period of research seeking successively better approximations to adequate classification and understanding.

In summary Grinker wrote:[18]

> Since psychiatric phenomena are social, to the extent
> that they arise from a social matrix; since they are
> precipitated, flourish, or decline under various social
> conditions, that is, they have an "epidemiology"; and
> since therapy depends to a degree on social and cul-
> tural factors, our interest in the contributions of the
> social sciences to the problem of etiology, although
> late and naive, is now growing. If we ever have any-
> thing to contribute to prevention, it will be through
> widespread social education at all levels. If our thera-
> peutic efforts are not to be limited to the few, there
> will have to be an increased interest in methods of
> understanding and eventually of treating the many,
> based on, but not simply a direct extension of our
> understanding of the individual. For these purposes
> education of psychiatrists will require extensive
> broadening, if not to widen the extent of their func-
> tions, at least to facilitate the cooperation of psychiatry
> with psychology, sociology and anthropology.

Social turbulence seems to be increasing in severity and
frequency in the latter half of the twentieth century and
constitutes a potent cause of serious stress responses.[19]
According to Levy,[20] we are paying a high price for modern
society's demand for efficiency and productivity; a price
that involves profound disturbances in the endocrine systems, and even a decrease in peripheral circulatory phago-
cytes—a decrease that predisposes individuals to
overwhelming infection.[21] Difficult though this kind of research may be, it is necessary and hopefully it will become
increasingly important.

REFERENCES

1. Hamburg, D. A. An evolutionary perspective on human ag-
   gressiveness. In D. Offer & D. X. Freedman (Eds.), *Modern
   psychiatry and clinical research.* New York: Basic Books, 1972.

2. Parsons, T. Boundary relations between sociocultural and personality systems. In R. Grinker (Ed.), *Toward a unified theory of human behavior.* New York: Basic Books, 1956, p. 325.
3. Grinker, R. R., Sr. (Ed.) *Toward a unified theory of human behavior.* (2nd ed.) New York: Basic Books, 1967.
4. Spiegel, J. P. Comparison of psychological and group foci. In R. Grinker (Ed.), *Toward a unified theory of human behavior.* (2nd ed.) New York: Basic Books, 1967, p. 164.
5. Spiegel, J. P., & Bell, N. W. The family of the psychiatric patient. In S. Arieti (Ed.), *Handbook of American psychiatry.* Vol. I. New York: Basic Books, 1959.
6. Grinker, R. R., Sr., & Spiegel, J. P. *Men under stress* (paperback). New York: McGraw-Hill Book Co., 1963.
7. Sanford, N. *Self and society: social change and individual development.* New York: Atherton Press, 1966.
8. Grinker, R. R., Sr., MacGregor, H., Selen, K., Klein, A. & Kohrman, J. *Psychiatric social work: a transactional case book.* New York: Basic Books, 1961.
9. Thompson, L. *The secret of culture.* New York: Random House, 1969.
10. Levy, L., & Rowitz, L. *The ecology of mental disorder.* New York: Behavioral Publications, 1973.
11. Zubin, J. On the power of models. *Journ. of Personality,* 1952, **20,** 430–439.
12. Cottle, T. J. L. *The prospect of youth.* Boston: Little Brown & Co., 1972.
13. Minuchin, A. *Families and family therapy: a structural approach.* Cambridge: Harvard University Press, 1974.
14. Faris, R. E. L. & Dunham, H. W. *Social theory and mental disorder.* Detroit: Wayne State University, 1959.
15. Hollingshead, A. B., & Redlich, F. C. *Social class and mental illness.* New York: John Wiley & Sons, 1958.
16. Cooper, B. & Morgan, H. C. *Epidemiological psychiatry.* Springfield, Ill.: Charles C. Thomas, 1973.
17. Clausen, J. A. The sociology of mental illness. In R. K. Merton, L. Broom, & L. S. Coltrell, Jr. (Eds.), *Sociology today.* New York: Basic Books, 1959.
18. Grinker, R. R., Sr. Goals for the future of American psychiatry. *Mount Sinai Journal of Medicine,* 1971, **38,** 226–242.

19. Cook, S. W. (Ed.) *Research methods in social relations.* Vols. 1 & 2. New York: Dryden Press, 1951.
20. Levy, L. Stress, distress and psychosocial stimuli. *Occupational Mental Health,* 1973, **3,** 2.
21. Palmbach, J., Froberg, I., Granstrom, G., Goren-Karlsson, C., Levi, L., & Unger, P. Stress and the human granulocyte. phagocytosis and turnover. *Reports from the Laboratory for Clinical Stress Research.* (Stockholm, Sweden), Dec., 1973, #34.

XI

Stress: Adaptation, Defenses, Coping and Disease

These words denote a large area of research of greatest significance for contemporary psychiatry. Coping and adaptation were the subjects of a recent multidisciplinary conference at Stanford University and a book edited by Coelho *et al.*[1] summarizes the literature to date.

We should accept the fact that "stress" as a generalized term is applicable only to universal catastrophes. Otherwise, the word stress should be utilized only when the individual family or group responds to a stimulus that meaningfully threatens the integrity of those to whom it is applied. "Adaptation" is a general biological term; "defense" stems from psychoanalysis; and "coping" generically includes these terms and others that will be discussed. In essence, the maintenance of self-esteem, a sense of human dignity, a sense of group belonging, and a feeling of being useful to others all seem to contribute significantly to survival in both physical and psychological terms. (Hamburg)[2]

Selye is one of the modern pioneers in stress research who has extended both theory and laboratory studies. He stated recently that stress cannot be defined, and I agree, because it has personal meaning. "Everybody knows what stress is but nobody knows what it is." Furthermore, "Complete freedom from stress is death." In other words, conflict is the essence of life. In his recent review, Selye[3] outlined his General Adaptation Syndrome in three stages that correspond to increased strain: 1) alarm; 2) resistance; and 3) exhaustion. The third stage represents the presence of diseases of adaptation which are individualized; in other words, they are personal readjustments or responses. The biological mechanisms involved in the mechanisms of adaptation are nervous, immunological or phagocytic and hormonal. Selye has carefully studied the activities of the hypothalamus, the sympathetic-adrenomedullary systems, the hypothyseal-adreno-cortical system and the activity of the thyroid gland. When long-continued and repeated stress-responses occur, organic systems reveal wear and tear and morphological changes.

For many years we were under the illusion that numerous psychosomatic diseases occurred in people in whom feelings and verbal and behavioral reactions were inhibited. Specific stresses evoked autonomic innervations as the sole response because these people could not express themselves in any other way. They were predisposed personalities.[4] Long-continued autonomic innervations converted dysfunctions in appropriate organs to morphologic changes and irreversible disease. For example, it was believed that frustrated dependency increased secretory activity of the stomach, ending in peptic ulcer. Repressed anger was supposed to culminate in the corresponding autonomic responses, producing fluctuating and then permanent hypertension. Unfortunately, these patterned responses were not confirmed by careful clinical scrutiny. The specific repressed emotional state did not correlate with the physiological results, and psychosomatic responses were not faithful to the stimuli.

When we were convinced that the enthusiastically received breakthrough could not be verified, it was necessary to restudy the effect of stress-stimuli on feelings and their physiological concomitants. To summarize briefly, we found that anxiety, anger and depression (and even intense pleasure) evoked adrenocortical responses of the same order as did any generalized emotional turbulence. Secondly, the emotional and physiological concomitants as resultants of stressful situations were specific for individuals. Thus it became clearer that specificity was not on the causal side of the chain of the events but on the resultant side.[5] Furthermore, the stimulus has to be personally meaningful to the subject. Thus we have to speak of stress-stimuli or situations, and specific stress responses (cf. Chapter VI).

Some stress responses seem to be part of man's evolutionary history and related to environments long since past, some associated with problems of development and others are related to current social and environmental changes. The research questions then become clearer: how does man adapt, defend or cope with these problems that arise during various phases of the lifecycle?

> The following are examples of common stressful experiences that have been emphasized in recent behavioral research and clinical discussions: separations from parents in childhood; displacement by siblings; childhood experiences of rejection; illness and injuries in childhood; illness and death of parents; severe illness and injuries of the adult years; the initial transition from home to school; puberty; later school transitions, e.g., from grade school to junior high school and from high school to college; competitive graduate education; marriage; pregnancy, menopause; necessity for periodic moves to a new environment; retirement; rapid technological and social change; wars and threats of wars; migration; acculturation; and social mobility. (Hamburg).[2]

There are of course individual differences in predispositions, responses and adaptations. These include previous levels of anxiety-proneness and ego involvement, commitment and goals in life. Avoidance and thereby reduction of information is one primitive mode of defense, but there are many others including social adaptation, seeking of new information, finding new friends and social groups, and new strategies appropriate to the attained age group.

Everyone needs to maintain a positive self-image and self-respect, as well as participation in a supporting social group and sufficient time for reappraisal of the infered dangerous situation. For these functions a person is prepared in early infancy by maternal protection and the support of a balance between autonomy and the ability to use help. The human child and adolescent have developmental time for learning by observation, imitation and exploration of their capacity for mastery. Later in life, rapid social and technological changes make coping more difficult. Cultural instructions and support from society become more ambiguous.

Moos[1] identifies three particular purposes for which further development of assessment techniques would be especially useful: 1) The possibility of altering coping strategies experimentally through interventions such as modeling and information-feedback; 2) The possibility of balancing costs and benefits of different coping strategies through intermediate and long time spans (months or years); 3) The possibility of understanding major cultural differences in coping behavior by developing techniques that have cross-cultural comparability.[6]

The work of Lazarus[1] touches on the sometimes unappreciated difficulty with a dichotomous classification between intrapsychic response and direct action response (mainly interpersonal). Bridging categories are needed, since responses to threat in fact typically involve an interplay between intrapsychic mechanisms and direct actions

In the last century the mind-body unity has interested many scientists from several disciplines.[9] There have been many attempts to develop unitary theories. Whyte's[10] phrase "unity in diversity and continuity in change" indicates personality with freedom of choice combined with generally acceptable social patterns of behavior. In Chapter II, Henry Holland's[11] statement of 1852 was quoted. So now we return to the so-called psychosomatic diseases (cf. Chapter VII).

For the last 30 years we have used the term "psychosomatic"—which seems to indicate a dichotomy more than it does a unity.[9] Nevertheless, this word is now imbedded in our language and firmly established in our literature. Is generally used to indicate a disease in which psychological factors are important but, as Engel[12] states, all bodily functions are unitary and psychosomatic. We seem most interested in and grasp more easily the unitary concepts of so-called psychosomatic medicine.[13] In fact, thousands of papers, many books and several periodicals devoted to this subject.

As we have briefly summarized investigations into stress-responses, defenses and coping devices in the hope that a better understanding of so-called psychosomatic disorders may result, we have been handicapped by the fact that our experiments can only be conducted on humans in a restricted laboratory space comparable to an animal cage, and for a brief period time. Such conditions are dissimilar to the free field which animals roam and humans live, and far short the time-span needed for the development of human illness. For such an understanding we should know a great deal about the human life-cycle since significant stimuli, stress and coping responses, adaptations, health and illness vary with phases of the cycle. One banal example; the homeostatic range of the is so wide that the sick child may appear to be

upon the environment. At least two such bridging concepts appear to be useful in much stress research: 1) the processes of appraisal and reappraisal described by Lazarus; 2) the processes of seeking and utilizing information described by Hamburg and Adams.[2]

An important suggestion implicit in the paper of Lazarus et al., and explicit in the work of Lois Murphy[1] and Beatrix Hamburg,[1] is the desirability of studying coping responses in terms of the stages of human development. The Lazarus experiments are cross-sectional, but similar experiments can be conducted at different age levels, in different eras of development and even in various field situations. In particular, the combination of experimental and field methods deserves further attention. Unfortunately, some kinds of adaptation, such as social deviance (delinquency) or even schizophrenic withdrawal, have a high cost.

Research on coping behavior emphasizes processes of human problem-solving in the direction of adaptive change. It brings into focus transactions of individuals or groups that are effective in meeting the requirements or utilizing the opportunities of specific environments. It highlights possibilities for enhancing the competence of individuals through developmental attainments, including ways of learning from exceptionally difficult circumstances. It is also beginning to suggest ways in which such stressful circumstances may be modified to diminish human suffering.

One of our residents has been engaged in studying "pleasure," which he equates with successful coping or mastery; the basis of ego growth through conflict. In a personal communication Dr. Fred Levin categorizes pleasure into phases: 1) pleasure through satisfaction of primary needs; 2) mastery of anxiety based on internal and external dangers; and 3) mastery of complex meanings and values (existential). Pleasure results from these stages of mastery which are, however, never completely successful.

The study of adaptation links the biological sciences, the social sciences and the clinical professions. The findings and implications of these studies are beginning to be useful in psychotherapy, counseling, rehabilitation, preventive intervention and education. Much, however, remains to be done in providing dependable information within the framework that has been constructed by workers in this field. We need to know more about the different personality structures that are associated with various forms of coping.

New information about coping patterns under specified conditions could benefit both individuals and institutions challenged by crises of social change. Such information, respecting the nature of human biology and the nature of social systems, could both help individuals acquire coping skills and assist institutions in anticipating typical or recurring coping exigencies.

Granted that there are biogenic, inherited or constitutional factors behind the development of the two major diseases in psychiatry—manic-depressive illness and schizophrenia—patients who become psychotic are, in all their ranges, attempting to cope with their innate dispositions and with the stresses impinging on them.[7]

> We assume that 1) a diatheses-stress model conforms to the data as we know them: life challenges ranging from serious illnesses or structural anomalies in infancy to narcissistic injuries are necessary to precipitate a predisposed (schizotaxic) individual into an overt schizophrenia and possibly eventually into psychosis, given the proper environmental field (Grinker).[7]

We shall discuss the problems of schizophrenia in Chapter XIII.

The adequacy of the coping process is not limited to the serious psychiatric diseases, but extends to degrees of

physical health and physical disease. This involves t' verbal "mind-body" problem that has fascinated , phers since antiquity, especially Aristotle. We separate mind and body on the basis of ego or distinctions.[8] Reality is what we perceive, which meaningful by virtue of the projections we imp perceptions—projections that are dependent dividual needs, experiences, frustrations and

> When we turn our attention to coping me related to continuous threats or repetitive ex of similar kind we enter the field of char personality and deal with health or normal hand and proneness to illness and dise other. The psychiatrist, true enough, has most exclusively on psychopathology ar recently neglected the normal or healthy deed is this since this therapeutic effort health and return the sick to the utopia mality.
>
> It would take us far afield to discus now being conducted on normal your clites) or modal adolescents or the va cal "sets" that are considered as norr from several hypotheses a few gene made. Various types of mental hea not only on drive derivatives, psy and their solutions, but also on sp factors. The capacity or role re necessary environments may resu nevertheless stable psychologica style searches for its appropria there is comfort and health. W stress-responses leading to p and physical disease. Thus t defenses and stress-suscep known about the organism this, statistical statements a meaningless.[5]

dying one hour and completely recovered the next. The aged may give little somatic evidence of serious illness and expire quickly. Certainly the psychosomatic and psychiatric problems vary greatly with phases of the life-cycle (Grinker).[14]

Alexander,[4] who pioneered the specificity hypotheses (later abandoned), which postulated that a specific repressed emotion is causally involved in a specific disease, has defined seven conditions as psychosomatic. These are outlined below with their supposed psychogenic components:

1. Bronchial asthma—threatened detachment from the mother;
2. Rheumatoid arthritis—difficulty with aggressive hostile impulses;
3. Ulcerative colitis—lost hope that tasks involving responsibilities can be accomplished;
4. Essential hypertension—struggle with asserting self;
5. Neurodermatitis—hunger for love as demonstrated by stroking;
6. Hyperthyroidism—fear of biological death;
7. Peptic ulcer—frustration of dependent and oral desires.

Despite Minuchen's[15] statement that psychosomatic diseases lack a conceptual model, more than enough investigators have attempted to devise models. Few people believe exclusively in the linear model—that a psychological conflict *causes* a physical disease. Minuchen uses the family model, evaluating it as overprotective, rigid and lacking forms for conflict-resolution—thus using the child, who is field-dependent, as a scapegoat. Mirsky[14] uses a constitutional plus social stress model for peptic ulcer; that is, a constitutional propensity toward increased pepsinogen secretion plus frustrating social events. Wolf[16] uses specificity to stressful life situations, Ruesch[17] writes about infantile personalities with problems in communication. Dunbar writes almost exclusively about constitution and Alexander,[4] Alexander, French and Pollock,[18] and Groen[19] use a psychodynamic model. Spiegel[9] used a transactional model, and Grinker[20] very early used a field concept. Grace and Graham[21] consider psychological attitudes most responsible for specific diseases. Spitz[22] believes early infantile experiences are important for future health.

Many correlations between specific psychological and specific somatic processes have been made but these now seem simple minded. Here are some of the single factors that have been used as explanatory concepts. These include hereditary constitution, birth injuries, organic diseases of infancy which increase the vulnerability of certain organs,[23] nature of infant care (weaning habits, toilet training, sleeping arrangements, etc.), accidental physical traumatic experiences of infancy and childhood,[24] emotional climate of family and specific personality traits of parents and siblings, later physical injuries, later emotional experiences in intimate personal and occupational relations.[25] These factors in different proportions are of etiological significance in all diseases. The psychosomatic point of view added the psychological factors to the other factors, which have long been given exclusive attention in medicine. Only the consideration of all these categories and their interaction can give a complete etiological picture.[26]

It is interesting that investigators working in the psychosomatic field write and speak loudly of the totality of the whole man, yet limit their work to small segments. There is a vast difference between rigorous biochemical and physiological research correlated with sloppy psychological anecdotes.[27] Certainly psychoanalytic studies are subjective and stereotyped and interviews in depth can confirm any desired theoretical point of view. The best we can hope for at this time is to consider psychosomatic as a mode of approach, but Alexander[4] belies even this when he differentiates between hysterical conversion symptoms and vegetative neuroses even though both involve both somatic and sympathetic nervous systems. As most of those involved in this problem will agree, there is a large amount of speculation but little data. If all levels of the organism are involved we need a common language for the totality.

Depending on the focus of interest, we need methods to ascertain the emotional deficiency suffered by infants, the degree of felt-separation from the mother, the temperament of the child that influences his subsequent behavior. But readers of the current literature complain that it is either too psychoanalytic or too biological or too social.

It is difficult to outline the principles of research on the neuroses. The discipline of psychoanalysis has probably been the main contributor to understanding their function-structure and psychogenesis, although psychoanalytic thinking has rarely been systematized in any fashion. One or a few case reports are still the subject matter of most publications and monotonous references to what Freud wrote are as yet the major contents of the written material. We recognize that one of Freud's major principles, conflict, is the source of anxiety against which the individual defends himself so that the entire field is designated as the "defense neuroses." Yet the vast psychoanalytic literature deals with explanations of the individual's historical experiential events to explain the specific symptoms which cover a wide range within each diagnostic class. It seems clear that little further may be gained from our understanding of neuroses by the clinical psychoanalytic approach, great though that contribution was originally.

The natural question for research is: can other methods, using the principles of other disciplines,[2] be applied to extend our etiological approach? This question applies to the classes of neuroses, personal and character neuroses, delinquency, etc. We can easily understand that all humans bear neurotic traits based on conflict and defense; man, as the end-product of a fantastic evolutionary pressure, is neurotic as a matter of course in that he struggles with conflicts between his animal drives and their pressures, which are controlled by the old brain, and his humanist, civilized, social and cultural achievements—which are regulated by his neopallium. Such strife between the two sides of his being engenders conflict which is expressed as anxiety, anger and depression. He defends against these by appropriate defensive lifestyles, but he usually survives without undue inner turmoil and with various degrees of social competence. His "normality" is thus a type of defense against his conflicts.

At a certain level, inner discomfort and difficulties in coping with social standards and cultural values may reach a threshold at which defenses assume quantitative values that mark him as being overtly "sick." We then diagnose him as being neurotic, classified as to the defenses he emphasizes. These defenses include obsessive, compulsive and phobic behaviors, as well as neurotic depression, schizoid withdrawal, deliquency, etc. Some of these neuroses are perceived as struggles against some extraneous and strange influence. Others, such as the character and personality neuroses, are long-standing and ego-syntonic, marking lifestyles that are fixed and difficult to reverse. The best proof that the formula "conflict, anxiety, neurosis" has some validity is that when a therapist weakens the defenses, rather than strengthens them, in order to expose the major conflict, he is confronted by the underlying anxiety.

It is interesting that before Freud's contribution of the concepts of symptom, inhibition and anxiety, psychiatrists thought that neuroses were attributable to constitutional factors. Freud agreed that constitutional factors were significant, but abandoned them because the therapist, then, could do nothing about them; he could, however, help the sufferer by increasing controls or by attempting to resolve the anxieties.

upon the environment. At least two such bridging concepts appear to be useful in much stress research: 1) the processes of appraisal and reappraisal described by Lazarus; 2) the processes of seeking and utilizing information described by Hamburg and Adams.[2]

An important suggestion implicit in the paper of Lazarus *et al.*, and explicit in the work of Lois Murphy[1] and Beatrix Hamburg,[1] is the desirability of studying coping responses in terms of the stages of human development. The Lazarus experiments are cross-sectional, but similar experiments can be conducted at different age levels, in different eras of development and even in various field situations. In particular, the combination of experimental and field methods deserves further attention. Unfortunately, some kinds of adaptation, such as social deviance (delinquency) or even schizophrenic withdrawal, have a high cost.

Research on coping behavior emphasizes processes of human problem-solving in the direction of adaptive change. It brings into focus transactions of individuals or groups that are effective in meeting the requirements or utilizing the opportunities of specific environments. It highlights possibilities for enhancing the competence of individuals through developmental attainments, including ways of learning from exceptionally difficult circumstances. It is also beginning to suggest ways in which such stressful circumstances may be modified to diminish human suffering.

One of our residents has been engaged in studying "pleasure," which he equates with successful coping or mastery; the basis of ego growth through conflict. In a personal communication Dr. Fred Levin categorizes pleasure into phases: 1) pleasure through satisfaction of primary needs; 2) mastery of anxiety based on internal and external dangers; and 3) mastery of complex meanings and values (existential). Pleasure results from these stages of mastery which are, however, never completely successful.

The study of adaptation links the biological sciences, the social sciences and the clinical professions. The findings and implications of these studies are beginning to be useful in psychotherapy, counseling, rehabilitation, preventive intervention and education. Much, however, remains to be done in providing dependable information within the framework that has been constructed by workers in this field. We need to know more about the different personality structures that are associated with various forms of coping.

New information about coping patterns under specified conditions could benefit both individuals and institutions challenged by crises of social change. Such information, respecting the nature of human biology and the nature of social systems, could both help individuals acquire coping skills and assist institutions in anticipating typical or recurring coping exigencies.

Granted that there are biogenic, inherited or constitutional factors behind the development of the two major diseases in psychiatry—manic-depressive illness and schizophrenia—patients who become psychotic are, in all their ranges, attempting to cope with their innate dispositions and with the stresses impinging on them.[7]

> We assume that 1) a diatheses-stress model conforms to the data as we know them: life challenges ranging from serious illnesses or structural anomalies in infancy to narcissistic injuries are necessary to precipitate a predisposed (schizotaxic) individual into an overt schizophrenia and possibly eventually into psychosis, given the proper environmental field (Grinker).[7]

We shall discuss the problems of schizophrenia in Chapter XIII.

The adequacy of the coping process is not limited to the serious psychiatric diseases, but extends to degrees of

physical health and physical disease. This involves the pro-
verbial "mind-body" problem that has fascinated philosophers since antiquity, especially Aristotle. We cannot
separate mind and body on the basis of ego or nonego
distinctions.[8] Reality is what we perceive, which becomes
meaningful by virtue of the projections we impose on our
perceptions—projections that are dependent on our individual needs, experiences, frustrations and successes.

> When we turn our attention to coping mechanisms
> related to continuous threats or repetitive experiences
> of similar kind we enter the field of character and
> personality and deal with health or normality on one
> hand and proneness to illness and disease on the
> other. The psychiatrist, true enough, has focused al-
> most exclusively on psychopathology and until very
> recently neglected the normal or healthy. Strange in-
> deed is this since this therapeutic effort is to facilitate
> health and return the sick to the utopian stage of nor-
> mality.
>
> It would take us far afield to discuss the researches
> now being conducted on normal young adults (homo-
> clites) or modal adolescents or the various psychologi-
> cal "sets" that are considered as normal. Nevertheless,
> from several hypotheses a few generalizations may be
> made. Various types of mental health are contingent
> not only on drive derivatives, psychological conflicts
> and their solutions, but also on special environmental
> factors. The capacity or role repertoires to fit into
> necessary environments may result in non-creative but
> nevertheless stable psychological equilibria. Thus life-
> style searches for its appropriate background. With it
> there is comfort and health. Without it there is strain,
> stress-responses leading to psychological regression
> and physical disease. Thus to understand coping or
> defenses and stress-susceptibility more must be
> known about the organism's past preparation. For
> this, statistical statements about small groups become
> meaningless.[5]

In the last century the mind-body unity has interested many scientists from several disciplines.[9] There have been many attempts to develop unitary theories. Whyte's[10] phrase "unity in diversity and continuity in change" indicates personality with freedom of choice combined with generally acceptable social patterns of behavior. In Chapter II, Henry Holland's [11] statement of 1852 was quoted. So now we return to the so-called psychosomatic diseases (cf. Chapter VII).

For the last 30 years we have used the term "psychosomatic"—which seems to indicate a dichotomy more than it does a unity.[9] Nevertheless, this word is now imbedded in our language and firmly established in our literature. It is generally used to indicate a disease in which psychological factors are important but, as Engel[12] states, all bodily functions are unitary and psychosomatic. We seem to be most interested in and grasp more easily the unitary concepts of so-called psychosomatic medicine.[13] In fact, thousands of papers, many books and several periodicals are devoted to this subject.

As we have briefly summarized investigations into stress-responses, defenses and coping devices in the hope that a better understanding of so-called psychosomatic disorders may result, we have been handicapped by the fact that our experiments can only be conducted on humans in a restricted laboratory space comparable to an animal cage, and for a brief period of time. Such conditions are dissimilar to the free field in which animals roam and humans live, and far short of the time-span needed for the development of human illness. For such an understanding we should know a great deal about the human life-cycle since significant stimuli, stress and coping responses, adaptations, health and illness vary with phases of the cycle. Just one banal example; the homeostatic range of the child is so wide that the sick child may appear to be dying one hour and completely recovered the next. The aged may give little somatic evidence of serious illness and expire quickly. Certainly the psychosomatic and psychiatric problems vary greatly with phases of the life-cycle (Grinker).[14]

Alexander,[4] who pioneered the specificity hypotheses (later abandoned), which postulated that a specific repressed emotion is causally involved in a specific disease, has defined seven conditions as psychosomatic. These are outlined below with their supposed psychogenic components:

1. Bronchial asthma—threatened detachment from the mother;
2. Rheumatoid arthritis—difficulty with aggressive hostile impulses;
3. Ulcerative colitis—lost hope that tasks involving responsibilities can be accomplished;
4. Essential hypertension—struggle with asserting self;
5. Neurodermatitis—hunger for love as demonstrated by stroking;
6. Hyperthyroidism—fear of biological death;
7. Peptic ulcer—frustration of dependent and oral desires.

Despite Minuchen's[15] statement that psychosomatic diseases lack a conceptual model, more than enough investigators have attempted to devise models. Few people believe exclusively in the linear model—that a psychological conflict *causes* a physical disease. Minuchen uses the family model, evaluating it as overprotective, rigid and lacking forms for conflict-resolution—thus using the child, who is field-dependent, as a scapegoat. Mirsky[14] uses a constitutional plus social stress model for peptic ulcer; that is, a constitutional propensity toward increased pepsinogen secretion plus frustrating social events. Wolf[16] uses specificity to stressful life situations, Ruesch[17] writes about infantile personalities with problems in communication. Dunbar writes almost exclusively about constitution and Alexander,[4] Alexander, French and Pollock,[18] and Groen[19] use a psychodynamic model. Spiegel[9] used a transactional model, and Grinker[20] very early used a field concept. Grace and Graham[21] consider psychological attitudes most responsible for specific diseases. Spitz[22] believes early infantile experiences are important for future health.

Many correlations between specific psychological and specific somatic processes have been made but these now seem simple minded. Here are some of the single factors that have been used as explanatory concepts. These include hereditary constitution, birth injuries, organic diseases of infancy which increase the vulnerability of certain organs,[23] nature of infant care (weaning habits, toilet training, sleeping arrangements, etc.), accidental physical traumatic experiences of infancy and childhood,[24] emotional climate of family and specific personality traits of parents and siblings, later physical injuries, later emotional experiences in intimate personal and occupational relations.[25] These factors in different proportions are of etiological significance in all diseases. The psychosomatic point of view added the psychological factors to the other factors, which have long been given exclusive attention in medicine. Only the consideration of all these categories and their interaction can give a complete etiological picture.[26]

It is interesting that investigators working in the psychosomatic field write and speak loudly of the totality of the whole man, yet limit their work to small segments. There is a vast difference between rigorous biochemical and physiological research correlated with sloppy psychological anecdotes.[27] Certainly psychoanalytic studies are subjective and stereotyped and interviews in depth can confirm any desired theoretical point of view. The best we can hope for at this time is to consider psychosomatic as a mode of approach, but Alexander[4] belies even this when he differentiates between hysterical conversion symptoms and vegetative neuroses even though both involve both somatic and sympathetic nervous systems. As most of those involved in this problem will agree, there is a large amount of speculation but little data. If all levels of the organism are involved we need a common language for the totality.

Depending on the focus of interest, we need methods to ascertain the emotional deficiency suffered by infants, the degree of felt-separation from the mother, the temperament of the child that influences his subsequent behavior. But readers of the current literature complain that it is either too psychoanalytic or too biological or too social.

It is difficult to outline the principles of research on the neuroses. The discipline of psychoanalysis has probably been the main contributor to understanding their function-structure and psychogenesis, although psychoanalytic thinking has rarely been systematized in any fashion. One or a few case reports are still the subject matter of most publications and monotonous references to what Freud wrote are as yet the major contents of the written material. We recognize that one of Freud's major principles, conflict, is the source of anxiety against which the individual defends himself so that the entire field is designated as the "defense neuroses." Yet the vast psychoanalytic literature deals with explanations of the individual's historical experiential events to explain the specific symptoms which cover a wide range within each diagnostic class. It seems clear that little further may be gained from our understanding of neuroses by the clinical psychoanalytic approach, great though that contribution was originally.

The natural question for research is: can other methods, using the principles of other disciplines,[2] be applied to extend our etiological approach? This question applies to the classes of neuroses, personal and character neuroses, delinquency, etc. We can easily understand that all humans bear neurotic traits based on conflict and defense; man, as the end-product of a fantastic evolutionary pressure, is neurotic as a matter of course in that he struggles with conflicts between his animal drives and their pressures, which are controlled by the old brain, and his humanist, civilized, social and cultural achievements—which are regulated by his neopallium. Such strife between the two sides of his being engenders conflict which is expressed as anxiety, anger and depression. He defends against these by appropriate defensive lifestyles, but he usually survives without undue inner turmoil and with various degrees of social competence. His "normality" is thus a type of defense against his conflicts.

At a certain level, inner discomfort and difficulties in coping with social standards and cultural values may reach a threshold at which defenses assume quantitative values that mark him as being overtly "sick." We then diagnose him as being neurotic, classified as to the defenses he emphasizes. These defenses include obsessive, compulsive and phobic behaviors, as well as neurotic depression, schizoid withdrawal, deliquency, etc. Some of these neuroses are perceived as struggles against some extraneous and strange influence. Others, such as the character and personality neuroses, are long-standing and ego-syntonic, marking lifestyles that are fixed and difficult to reverse. The best proof that the formula "conflict, anxiety, neurosis" has some validity is that when a therapist weakens the defenses, rather than strengthens them, in order to expose the major conflict, he is confronted by the underlying anxiety.

It is interesting that before Freud's contribution of the concepts of symptom, inhibition and anxiety, psychiatrists thought that neuroses were attributable to constitutional factors. Freud agreed that constitutional factors were significant, but abandoned them because the therapist, then, could do nothing about them; he could, however, help the sufferer by increasing controls or by attempting to resolve the anxieties.

Now, however, a biogenetic, constitutional basis for severe neuroses has become a focus for research. Observations are being made on early evidences of constitutional differences which are at present not apparent in direct studies of the genes. Escalona[28] and others have made extensive observations on children during the early weeks of life, revealing differences in function and behavior that are possibly linked to the strength of later ego development; these studies have also revealed differing capacities to control drive strengths that predict overriding influences over ego functions.

Another focus is on direct observations of development independent of the maturational pace, but dependent on patterns of parenthood and accidental extraneous factors of infections, trauma, etc. From these investigations, predictions of subsequent degrees of neurotic imbalance may be made and appropriate early methods of primary prevention may be devised.

In sum, psychoanalytic investigations of conflict may be explanations, but the data is retrospective and fallible. The true essence of neurotic predispositions may be ascertained by direct observations of child development, a field shunned by most psychiatrists but valiantly exploited by child psychologists.

There are so many conceptual approaches to the relationship among the various biological and psychological processes constituting the human organism that only a general, field and unitary theory could encompass the whole. From Aristotle to the present, this notion has persisted, but is difficult to put into operation by methods that include all parts of the whole. Not only do techniques differ, but significant correlations among more than two are difficult to verify.

Anecdotal and systematic descriptions of growth, development, stress, trauma, defenses and coping devices produce such a vast array of indigestible data that one is tempted to leave the field and focus on more localized problems. Regression during disease to a more primitive state of the organism may require the study of a single dependent variable through states of development and back again. Anxiety is an example of how this may be done (cf. Chapter XIII).[29] Another example is the symbolic system[30] in its evolution and disintegration (cf. Chapter II).

It seems that it might be possible to recognize that there are some processes for which general commonality or systems' properties may be traced from their biological roots to their social flowering; provided, that is, that describable and understandable specific modifications, depending on the part of the system under the focus of observation, are also taken into account.

We can analyze a single function or process as an organizer of behavior that is recognizable as antecedent to known effects. If the process is not emphasized out of proportion, it has survival value; if it takes undue prominence, it leads to disintegration. We may view these properties with equanimity as respectable teleology. Then suppose we study this function as it becomes a part of various systems of organization and observe its relationship to the other parts of a system and to its whole.

Finally, we may study how it is involved in functions of each system in relation to other systems. Each of the following propositions involves separate operational procedures and different frames of reference. If these can be synthesized, a single building block for a unified theory may be at hand.

1. All functions of the living human organism, whether in health or illness, are psychosomatic.

2. All disturbances in human function are adaptive and involve multiple processes and causes.

3. Varying constellations of processes may find the same functional expression in a final common pathway.

4. The total human organism, in varying interrelationships with other organisms and the material world, and the part-functions of any single human organism are viewed as transactional processes among themselves.

5. Rather than utilizing the notion of psychic energy, we view relationships from the frame of reference of communications and the transmission of information. This is possible whether we are talking about social, psychological or somatic behavior.

6. The influence of strain on the organism differs with the phase of its developmental process or the state of regression at the time, and stress is the sum total of organismic response.

7. Heredity, constitution, strength of instinctual forces, life experiences with the first nuclear family and ever-extending social groups, precipitating factors, etc. are all important in the production of illness. Each has a place in the transacting field of strain and adaptation.

8. The organs that comprise the human body should not be isolated as single targets for a study of healthy function or illness for they are organized into open systems with highly permeable boundaries.[31/32] But as Freud[33] said in a personal communication 40 years ago, "That is the future of Medicine." By this he meant that some day the above principles will be ready for more exact study by improved methods. He was correct. We are still not ready.

REFERENCES

1. Coelho, G. V., Hamburg, D. A., Moos, R., & Randolph, P. (Eds.) *Coping and adaptation: a behavioral science bibliography.*

Washington, D.C.: National Institute of Mental Health, 1970. Also, *Coping and adaptation*. New York: Basic Books, 1974.

2. Hamburg, D. A., & Adams, J. A perspective on coping behavior: seeking and utilizing information in major transactions. *Arch. Gen. Psych.;* 1967, **17,** 277–284.

3. Selye, H. The evolution of the stress concept. *American Scientist,* 1973, **61,** 692–698. Also, Selye, H. *Stress without distress.* Philadelphia: J. B. Lippincott, 1974.

4. Alexander, F. *Psychosomatic medicine.* New York: Norton, 1950.

5. Grinker, R. R., Sr. *Psychosomatic research.* (2nd ed.) New York: Grove Press, 1961. Also Grinker, R. R., Sr. *Psychosomatic concepts.* (3rd ed). New York: Jason Aronson, 1974.

6. Kluckhohn, F., & Strodbeck, F. B. *Variations in value orientations.* Evanston, Ill.: Row-Peterson, 1963.

7. Grinker, R. R., Sr., & Holzman, P. S. Schizophrenic pathology in young adults. *Arch. Gen. Psych.,* 1973, **28,** 125–168.

8. Bertalanffy, L. V. Mind and body re-examined. *Journ. Humanistic Psychology,* Fall, 1966, 113–138.

9. Spiegel, J. P. *Transactions.* New York: Science House, 1971.

10. Whyte, L. L. *The next development in man.* New York: Henry Holt, 1948.

11. Holland, H. *Mental physiology.* London: Longmans, Brown, Green, & Longmans, 1852.

12. Engel, G. *Psychological development in health and disease.* Philadelphia: W. B. Saunders, 1962.

13. Cannon, W. *Wisdom of the body.* New York: W. W. Norton, 1963.

14. Grinker, R. R., Sr. Psychiatry and our dangerous world. In G. F. S. Heseltine (Ed.), *Psychiatric research in our changing world.* Amsterdam: Excerpta Medica, 1969.

15. Minuchin S., Baker, L., Rosman, B. L., Liebman, R., Milman, L., & Todd, T. C. Psychosomatic illness in children: a new conceptual model. Cambridge, Mass.: Harvard University Press, 1974.

16. Wolf, G. H. Life situations and stress in life stress and bodily disease: a formulation. *Proc. Assoc. Res. Nerv. Ment. Disease,* 1950, 29, 1059.

17. Ruesch, J. The infantile personality—the core problem of psychosomatic medicine. *Psychosomatic Medicine,* 1948, **10,** 134.

18. Alexander, F., French, T. M., & Pollack, G. H. *Psychosomatic specificity.* Vol. I. Chicago: *University of Chicago Press,* 1968.
19. Groen, J. Substitute theory of psychosomatic disease. *Journ. Psychosomatic Research,* 1957, **2,** 85–96.
20. Grinker, R. R., Sr., & Robbins, F. *Psychosomatic case book.* New York: Blakiston, 1954.
21. Grace, W. T., & Graham, D. T. Relationship of specific attitudes and emotions to certain bodily diseases. *Psychosomatic Med.,* 1952, **14,** 243–251.
22. Spitz, R. A. Relevancy of direct infant observations. *The Psychoanal. Study of the Child,* 1950, **5,** 66–75.
23. Grinker, R. R., Sr. The effect of infantile disease on ego patterns. *Amer. Journ. Psychiatry,* 1953, **110,** 290–295.
24. Bowlby, J. *Attachment and loss.* Vol. I. New York: Basic Books, 1969.
25. Basowitz, H., Korchin, S. J., Persky, H., & Grinker, R. R., Sr. *Anxiety and stress.* New York: Blakiston, 1955.
26. Benedek, T. *Studies in psychosomatic medicine.* New York: Ronald Press, 1952.
27. Roessler, R., & Greenfield, N. S. (Eds.) *Physiological correlates of psychological disorder.* Madison, Wis.: University of Wisconsin Press, 1962.
28. Escalona, S., & Heider, S. M. *Prediction and outcome.* New York: Basic Books, 1959.
29. Grinker, R. R., Sr. Anxiety as a significant variable for a unified theory of human behavior. *Arch. Gen. Psych,* 1959, **1,** 537–546.
30. Grinker, R. R., Sr. Symbolism and general systems theory. In W. Gray, F. J. Duhl, and N. D. Rizzo (Eds.), *General systems theory and psychiatry.* Boston: Little, Brown & Co. 1969.
31. Sahakian, W. S. (Eds.) *Psychopathology today.* Itasca, Ill.: F. E. Peacock, 1970.
32. Witkower, E. D., & Cleghorn, R. A. (Eds.) *Recent developments in psychosomatic medicine.* Philadelphia: J. B. Lippincott, 1960.
33. Grinker, R. R., Sr. Freud and Medicine. *Bull. New York Academy of medicine,* 1956, **32,** 878–886.

XII

Clinical Research

The focus of research in psychiatry is the human subject whose suffering is the major interest of mental health specialists. Without a profound understanding of human psychopathology, all other disciplines such as genetics, biochemistry, sociology, etc., dangle free without support of stable referents. Yet our ability to diagnose and classify mental disorders is still primitive and we have yet to answer satisfactorily the question "what?"

Clinical research—excluding psychoanalysis, which has its own method—has four important tools: observations of behavior, the interview, questionnaires and psychological tests. In a general sense, it is these techniques that justify including clinical research as one of the behavioral sciences.[1] It may seem that these tools are possessed by anyone with eyes, ears and a capacity for abstraction, but this is far from true.

Psychiatrists are notoriously poor observers of behavior.[2] Their training has usually concentrated on listening to verbal statements for the purpose of understanding covert meanings. Clinical psychologists, on the other hand, do observe well, and when reporting test-results describe in great detail the behaviors of their subjects.

Conducting interviews requires both the patience to listen in an unstructured system of communications and the ability to subsequently conduct structured interrogations that reflect a knowledge of those sequences of thinking and feeling that are appropriate to the goal of the research. Interviewing is a delicate tool that requires complete familiarity with its goal and continuous use in order for the interviewer to acquire a body of experience and sensitivity to the patient's feelings and defensive maneuvers. This skill is not easily perfected and, like any instrument, it needs constant calibration.

Questionnaires are not simple instruments that can be put together quickly. They need considerable thought to be sure that the items are directly pertinent to the information sought. Furthermore, each word needs to be carefully studied to be sure that it has a universally and well-understood single meaning. For example, a question asked college students was worded: "Was your mother concerned about . . . ?" The word concern was interpreted by some as *worried* and by others as benign *interest*. To avoid such indefinite questions the questionnaire should be given a liberal pretest.

Psychiatrists are dubious about the use of psychological tests in research, since once a test has been *presumed* to tap a specific psychological resource, it is utilized forever more *as if* that specific goal has been validated. As a result, names of tests are floating around to be pulled into a research for purposes that they cannot fulfill. So, for example, the MMPI has numerous shortcomings, yet it is used because there is "nothing better." The same criticism applies to the I.Q. and the Rorschach tests and to many other rating scales that have poor reliability and validity; the same research could often be better done if nondirective interviews[3] were used instead. Measurements of intelligence and of personality as well as diagnosis of brain damage (organicity), should utilize tests, but should not forego interviews and questionnaires.

Questionnaires must be constructed to fit the goal of the research and cannot be borrowed. Such an instrument was devised by us in studying the predisposition of flying personnel[4] to the development of operational fatigue (war neuroses). Also, the most effective tests are devised by innovators. An example is the "stress tolerance test," a new projective technique utilizing both meaningful and meaningless stimuli, which furnished an objective measure of the war neurotics' degree of improvement.[5] Another special technique was devised to produce anxiety by perceptual distortion.[6]

The tools of clinical research, consisting of interviews, questionnaires and tests, are developed, calibrated and sharpened by investigators in the mental health field; these investigators consist of psychiatrists, clinical psychologists, social workers, anthropologists and sociologists. The latter two disciplines have their own methods and may engage in cooperative research with the first two. Social workers often function in an ancillary fashion with the other clinicians but rarely independently. But the main body of clinical research is carried on by psychiatrists and clinical psychologists who use the same tools. Despite their different backgrounds and training, we should not separate them but should consider them as unidisciplinary groups—as exemplified by the current partnership of Grinker and Holzman.[7]

One of the tools psychologists have proposed to delve into the depths of personality is hypnosis, about which, however, there is considerable uncertainty. Hilgard[8] states that there are major unknowns and disputes about the adequacy of the evidence garnered from various experiments.[9] Strangely, although hypnosis has been around for a long time, even as a direct precursor of psychoanalysis, the concept of hypnosis is still not clearly defined.

Rodnick[10] indicates that personality is the subject matter of psychology; and psychology, as a science, is strained in its relationship to other disciplines—except for medicine.

We would comment that psychophysiology, psychophysics and psychochemistry are theoretically close, but usually one part of these hybrid terms is neglected. Yet, for all somatic and psychological functions there seems to be a final common pathway.

Psychologists have, of course, interest in drive theories,[11] from which other psychopathological qualities are presumed to develop. So, for example, increased stimulus input acting on a heightened drive arousal would be accompanied by a low threshold for disorganization and stimulus generalization. Thus such an inadequately modulated system would require narrowed attention as a protective device to reduce input and avoid excessive excitation.

Psychologists in general, as well as clinical psychologists in particular, reveal their academic background despite their growing interest in human problems as a field for study. We do recognize that psychology is not the basic science for psychiatry in the sense that physiology is the basic science for medicine. But the concern for theory and constructs has split psychology into multiple schools detached with varying distances from empirical data. This they are overcoming by becoming more involved in psychiatric clinics and with psychiatric research partners. At the same time we need such constructs as Rimoldi's[12] innate logical structures, Piaget's[13] ontogeny of thought, Vigotsky's[14] development of inner speech as a problem of social psychology and Whorf's[15] studies on language, thought and reality.

Psychology is an extensive discipline, really a profession composed of many parts, just as is psychiatry. The earliest appearing branch was concerned with research, and that mostly on normal mental functioning. Following the lead of the psychiatric social workers, who were pressed into the roles of psychotherapists, clinical psychologists increased in number but never achieved the status of their scientific brethren in psychology, despite their common Ph.D. degree.

Psychiatrists in clinics were accustomed to ordering psychologists to perform psychological tests as if they were laboratory technicians; but gradually the clinical psychologist insisted on being a consultant to the psychiatrist both before and after his psychometric activities were carried out. It was not much later that the psychologist became an equal and integral part of the research team. Even so, he did, and still does, maintain an interest in formal theory, rigor and neatness in design. The clinical psychologist has lessened his degree of interest in specific tests for psychopathology of various types and relies more on the interview. In that sense, the psychiatrist also has learned greater skills in the details of the interview and their interpretations.

Psychiatry, as we have indicated in previous chapters, is a descendant of psychology and philosophy under the umbrella of medicine. The field has been under strong biological influence, which has been somewhat equalized and directed toward the humanities by the psychoanalytic intrusion of the last several decades. Its academic tradition is weak since medical education prepares the student for a medical therapeutic career. Further, graduate education is concentrated on diagnosis and treatment, with only a few candidates attaining career research fellowships.

Despite these differences in professional histories and in backgrounds of training, we include psychiatrists and psychologists on a parity in clinical research. Yet, even together, we frequently feel the need to include practitioners of other disciplines such as biochemists, physiologists, etc. in our work—as in our stress research or current schizophrenic programs. Or we ourselves may join other programs. In fact, we often end up being part of a multidisciplinary team.

Shakow,[16] a psychologist, has studied schizophrenia for most of his life—working with other disciplines, including physiology, psychophysiology, experimental psychology and clinical psychology. Out of these methods have come hypotheses such as "neophobia," variations of arousal levels, various abilities to maintain a "major set" giving rise to easy distraction and the use of a segmental set. These phenomena will later be described in a discussion of schizophrenia, where they are most prominent (Chapter XIII). Shakow also makes some interesting statements about variability in clinical research depending on the position and function of the observer. He enumerates the different types of observers as follows: the objective observer, the participant observer, the subjective observer and finally the self-observer of biases and expectancies.

Research in the field of psychiatry has certain built-in limitations, depending on the goal. The three major questions of what, how and why are concerned with diagnosis —classification, etiology and teleology. Each question utilizes different disciplines and methods. For example, research on the definition of the borderline syndrome or on delinquency is limited to focal segments of the entire field, which calls on the resources of few disciplines; research on schizophrenia, on the other hand, which we shall discuss later, involves extensive use of many disciplines and application of all the components of general systems theory.

Some research may be conducted in naturalistic settings, involving only subjects who are carrying on their usual behavior; this is true in anthropological and sociological investigations and in psychiatry as exemplified by Basowitz et al.[17] in their work on anxiety and stress. Other human investigations employ the experimental method such as the application of stress in an interview, or in viewing motion pictures with concomitant or subsequent biochemical, physiological or psychological tests. Many experimental designs such as the two mentioned above are now not feasible because of required "informed consent."

Another decision that has to be made concerns the use of cross-sectional versus longitudinal approaches but both may be employed in certain cases. The combination was used by Offer[18] in his study of normal adolescents and is being used in our schizophrenic program. Each approach (cross-sectional and longitudinal) has its place in psychiatric research, but the *what* question requires long-continued follow-up studies to control for spontaneous or life experienced changes in the syndrome and shifts in symptoms— as, for example, in the case of a schizophrenia that shifts from acute to chronic and chronic to terminal.

Follow-up studies in longitudinal research are necessary not only because of changes occuring in different phases of ontogenetic development, but because of shifting motivation of the subjects and alterations, depending on life-stresses, in patterns of defense and coping. In some conditions, outcome depends on the kind and quantity of external social support; as, for example, the differences in outcome between single family-less schizophrenics and those fully accepted and helped by concerned relatives and communities. The follow-up studies may be conducted by means of interviews, questionnaires, tests or all of them. The attrition or drop-out rate of subjects is often great, so the beginning number of subjects should be at least double those expected to cooperate to completion, and the follow-up tactics need to be aggressively pursued.

What kinds of controls are necessary? First, we need to use the same procedures on subjects suffering (as patients) with conditions other than the one under investigation. Secondly, we need so-called "normals" or "healthy" persons. These are both difficult to define and difficult to find. In fact, paid volunteers are often psychopathic. Grinker, Grinker and Timberlake[19] studied a group of young adult college students who were psychologically healthy and

Grinker and Werble[20] sent them questionnaires 14 years later finding them to be even healthier than at the time of the first study. This group of 134 (males only) is available for use by any interested investigator (cf. Chapter VII).

In clinical research as in other scientific endeavor tests for reliability and validity insure the legitimacy of the results, but these can only be expressed in probabalistic terms. The conclusions of the research may be expressed in the hard firm language of the obtained data, but they may also include new hypotheses and speculations as to their meaning, providing each is clearly defined as to what it stands for.

When we study a human being, unlike in the study of laboratory animals, we meet many uncontrollable factors that should at least be recognized. We know that the setting of the research is limited in time and that many experiences extraneous to this setting are not controllable, even in a hospital ward. What life crises are outside our knowledge? What spontaneous shifts in the disturbance occur? In the here-and-now interview or test procedure we obtain a sample of cognitive, affective and behavioral structures, but past histories indicating prior ego strength or predisposing factors are hard to elicit truthfully from the subject or his family.

When dealing with large samples of subjects in order to wipe out individual differences, a statistician should be included in the research team during the planning stages to prevent the possibility that the final result will be only the garbage that the computer abhors—and simply regurgitates as garbage in a different form. Sophisticated clinical research today demands more than simple correlational analyses. Instead we should use cluster analyses, principle component analyses and/or factor analyses. All these demand mathematical and statistical expertise that clinicians do not usually possess.

The statistical results should match closely with clinical experience. As clinicians, we have the responsibility of choosing which, among several possible groupings, are logically compatible with clinical experience and which have the optimum degree of discrimination for clinical practice. Very frequently a fit is achieved which could not have been possible by clinical scanning or statistical analysis alone.[21]

We frequently speak of psychiatric research as essentially concerned with ego functions as expressed in behaviors. But we rarely enumerate these hypothetical functions or translate them into observable and describable behaviors. Beres[22] enumerates ego functions under seven headings:

1. *Relation to Reality.* *a.*) Adaptation to reality depends upon the external demands or obstacles to need-satisfactions. The individual in action requires a repertoire of internalized social roles that he can play spontaneously and actions which on necessity he can devise (creatively) toward people, things and tasks. This means the capacity to grow, differentiate and integrate. *b.*) Reality-testing requires accuracy of perception, capacity to orient self in time and place, tolerance for ambiguity and judgment as to the differentiation between figure and ground (focusing). *c.*) Sense of reality is manifested by unobtrusive ordinary functions which differentiate self from others based on effective automatic recognition of the boundaries of self (identity). This involves an "ego feeling" which constitutes an effective awareness of self maintained over time (stability) which also resists diffusion or depletion.

2. *Regulation and Control of Drives.* This function concerns effective control of inner pressures which demands tolerance of frustration, anxiety and ambiguity. It depends on such tactics as detour-behavior, delay and sublimation.

3. *Object-Relations.* The ability to form such relations and to maintain their consistency notwithstanding ambivalences, rejections or frustrations.

4. *Cognitive Functions.* These include concentration, selective scanning, memory, abstraction and ability to avoid contamination by drive expressions.

5. *Defensive Functions.* Included are the various types of defenses appropriate to both inner and outer pressures, such as repression, reaction-formation, denial, withdrawal and adaptive or coping mechanisms.

6. *Autonomous Functions.* These cognitive functions are considered to be the "givens" of the conflict-free ego and include perception, intention (energy or will), intelligence and language capacity.

7. *Synthetic Functions.* An important capacity includes the ability to organize, to form gestalts and to compromise.

Behavior—verbal and nonverbal—is the basic data of scientific psychiatry. Behavior represents in actuality functions that have been allocated to a hypothetical ego; an ego which, on the one hand, filters perceptions and actions, and on the other, expresses reportable motivations, affects, defenses and compromises, employs symptoms and sublimations and demonstrates integrative capacities and disintegrative trends. We espouse a form of behavioral study that acknowledges the existence of unconscious mental processes and accepts introspection reported by verbal responses that subjects make under given conditions.

We can state the conceptual theory that ego-functions are the final common pathway for the expression of mentation at any level, no matter what technical means are adopted for their observation or in what situation—psychoanalysis or in a mental hospital nursing unit—they occur. Ego functions are expressed in behaviors which are observable and describable. The research task in defining a clinical syndrome is to observe well-defined aspects of behavior. Behaviors may be studied under five headings:[21]

1. *Outward behavior* used as measures of adaptation to reality, that is, the adaptation of the ego to people, environment and tasks.

2. *Perception* used as measures of reality-testing, sense of reality and some cognitive functions.
3. *Messages* used as measures of language capacity.
4. *Affects and defenses* used as measures of object-relations, regulation and control of drives and defensive functions.
5. *Synthesis* used as measures of capacity for problem-solving and organization.

Since the prime question in psychiatric clinical research is defining, both by inclusion and exclusion, what constitutes a clinical syndrome, we deal with patients who are getting some form of treatment. Many times the psychotherapist not only does not cooperate, but interferes with the research, so that, if possible, research and treatment should be separate functions. Certainly the "what" question cannot at this time be answered by the results of therapy.

One area of research for which the usual tools of clinical research are used is the family. Using the family as a focus instead of the individual, observations, interviews, tests and group tasks may clarify the systems of communications, and the power hierarchy, which crippled at least one of its members. This will be exemplified when we discuss schizophrenia, because as yet special family processes seem to be identifiable only for that disorder.[23]

Aside from the traditional theories developed by psychiatrists and psychologists, we are witnessing a number of mystical concepts that do not offer tools for research. They are phenomenological, dealing only with consciousness and a subjective frame of reference that cannot be altered by commands.[24] Among these theories are the existentialist ones that deal with "becoming," the personal construct theory of anticipation of events, the positive self-regard concepts, the "third force" of growth *as* safety and the search for security. These may be humanitarian in outlook, but they reject objectivity, reality and research.

A neglected area of research in psychiatry is concerned with development within and among the phases of the life-cycle. Certainly there is a patchwork quilt of theories of child development expressed in behavioral terms (Baldwin[25]). Piaget's[13] schemas of intelligence as action patterns leading to accommodation to the environment and internalized assimilation have been widely acclaimed, but his research is based on incomplete empirical data written in a style difficult to understand. Nurnberger[26] outlines the various serious nutritional, metabolic, infectious and environmental factors that influence future development. Early upsets at environmental changes in infancy may be predictive of later trouble, but the crying need in this field is for longitudinal studies. Offer's[18] studies of the teenager are systematic and methodologically sound, as contrasted with most other anecdotal reports of experiences of children, adolescents, young adults, adults and elderly—although the latter group has fared better at the hands of researchers than the other phases of life.

REFERENCES

1. Hamburg, D. (Ed.) *Psychiatry as a behavioral science.* Englewood Cliffs, N.J.: Prentice-Hall, 1970.
2. Grinker, R. R., Sr., Miller, J., Sabshin, M., Nunn, R., & Nunnally, J. C. *The phenomena of depressions.* New York: Hoeber, 1961.
3. Hoch, P. H., & Zubin, J. *Relation of psychological tests to reality.* New York: Grune & Stratton, 1952.
4. Grinker, R. R., Sr., Willerman, B., Bradley, A. D., & Fasttofsky, A. A study of psychological predisposition to the development of operational fatigue. *Amer. Journal of Orthopsych.,* 1946, **16,** 191–214.
5. Harrower, M. R., & Grinker, R. R., Sr. The stress tolerance test. *Psychosomatic Medicine,* 1946, **8,** 3–15.
6. Korchin, S., Basowitz, H., Grinker, R. R., Sr., Hamburg, D., Persky, H., Sabshin, M., Heath, H., & Board, F. Experience

of perceptual distortion as a source of anxiety. *A.M.A. Arch. of Neurol. and Psych.*, 1958, **80**, 98–113.

7. Grinker, R. R., Sr., & Holzman, P. S. Schizophrenic pathology in young adults. *Arch. Gen. Psychiatry.*, 1973, **28**, 168–175.

8. Hilgard, E. R. The domain of hypnosis: with some comments on alternative paradigms. *American Psychologist*, 1973, **28**, 972–983.

9. Royce, J. R. (Ed.) *Psychology and the symbol.* New York: Random House, 1965.

10. Rodnick, E. H. Clinical psychology, psychopathology and research on schizophrenia. In S. Koch (Ed.), *Psychology: a study of a science.* Vol. 15. New York: McGraw-Hill, 1963.

11. Epstein, S., & Coleman, M. Drive theories of schizophrenia. *Psychosomatic Medicine*, 1970, **32**, 113–140.

12. Rimoldi, H. S. Thinking and language. *Arch. Gen. Psych.*, 1967, **17**, 568–576.

13. Piaget, J. *Origins of intelligence in children.* New York: International Universities Press, 1951.

14. Vigotsky, L. S. *Thought and language.* Cambridge, Mass.: M.I.T. Press, 1962.

15. Whorf, B. L. *Language, thought and reality.* Cambridge, Mass.: M.I.T. Press, 1964.

16. Shakow, D. Some observations on the psychology (and some fewer, on the biology) of schizophrenia. *Journ. Nerv. Ment. Dis.*, 1971, **153**, 300–316.

17. Basowitz, H., Korchin, S. J., Persky, H., & Grinker, R. R., Sr. *Anxiety and stress.* New York: Blakiston, 1955.

18. Offer, D. *The psychological world of the teen-ager.* New York: Basic Books, 1969.

19. Grinker, R. R., Sr., Grinker, R. R., Jr., & Timberlake, J. Mentally healthy young males (homoclites). *Arch. Gen. Psych.*, 1962, **6**, 405–453.

20. Grinker, R. R., Sr., & Werble, B. Mentally healthy young males (homoclites) 14 years later. *Arch. Gen. Psych.* 1974, **30**, 701–704.

21. Grinker, R. R., Sr., Werble, B., & Drye, R. C. *The borderline syndrome.* New York: Basic Books, 1968.

22. Beres, D. Structure and function in psychoanalysis. *Int. Journ. Psychoanal.*, 1965, **46**, 53–63.

23. Jackson, D. D. (Ed.) *The etiology of schizophrenia.* New York: Basic Books, 1960.
24. Brewster-Smith, M. The phenomological approach in personality theory: some critical remarks. *Journ. Abnorm. and Soc Psychology,* 1950, **45,** 516–522.
25. Baldwin, A. L. *Theories of child development.* New York: John Wiley, 1968.
26. Nurnberger, J. I. *Biological and environmental determinants of early development.* Baltimore: Williams & Wilkins, 1973.

XIII

Developing an Integrated Theory: The Example of Schizophrenia

We utilize a systems approach to psychiatry;[1,2] that is, we deal with it is as a conglomerate science composed of a variable number of parts (see Chapter III). Which of these parts we use is a matter of choosing among the several available perspectives. For example, the "parts" may be the various contributory disciplines from biogenetics to sociology. Or we may choose the ontogenetic frame of reference, using thereby the maturational and developmental phases of the lifecycle from infancy to old age. But whichever point of view the observer adopts, he is still working in terms of a "system," e.g., a model of relationship in action viewed from different perspectives depending on the position of the observer.[3]

Then there is another set of systems—the systems by which the human person maintains his integrity. These systems are held together and integrated by a supraordinated regulatory or control function that is evolved during development. When this function loses its grip on its physical or mental control, because of excessive strain or disease, dissolution in the Jacksonian sense occurs (or regression as defined by Freudian psychoanalysis), i.e., the parts are released from control and two sets of phenomena appear.[4] One set is negative, in that some ego- or self-functions are lost. The other set appears as a positive expression of previously inhibited part-functions.

The questions then, in relation to this system collapse, are *"What* is happening?" *"How* is it happening?" and *"Why* is it happening?" Psychiatry's function is to integrate the clinical data that apply to these questions and to use all the parts of the psychiatric system to contribute the answers[5] when techniques are available. Unfortunately, answers to even the first question are still uncertain because, after almost a century, our systems of diagnoses and nosological classification remain inadequate. This has happened largely because nonclinical research psychiatry and clinical psychiatry have tended to go off in different directions, instead of working together. A nonclinician, for example, will often come up with a piece of information that has no application to a specific clinical entity. The clinician, unable to use the information, ignores it, and thus, instead of filling in the puzzle together, the two parts of the system work in a vacuum. Investigators in schizophrenia, for example, who are becoming increasingly aware that we are not sure of what the schizophrenias are, tend to split off in isolation; one group indulges in so-called reductionism on the biological side, and the other group on the opposite pole indulges in "humanism." It is for these reasons that clinical psychiatry should concentrate more on research to bring together these two perspectives and elucidate the *what* question.

In this chapter I shall attempt to describe how the different parts of the psychiatric system can be integrated as is demonstrated in work in the schizophrenias. We found when we organized our schizophrenia program that it could be well handled by an extensive systems approach in longitudinal research, bolstered by sophisticated statistical analyses. Thus the contributions of the clinical, biological and statistical perspectives could all be brought into play to develop a unified theory.

THE "WHAT:" CLASSIFICATION, SYMPTOMATOLOGY

The general usefulness, reliability and validity of psychiatric diagnosis with special reference to schizophrenia evoke the false contrast between the medical or disease-entity model and the social model applied to psychological and behavioral deviance. Since classifications are the first, albeit tottering, steps toward a scientific psychiatry, it matters not at all whether the labels applied are disease, disorder, deviance, faulty behavior, or even degrees of faulty education or stupidity. From whichever stance the situation is viewed, diagnosis has become a necessity for progress in every aspect of the large, extended field that we call psychiatry. If we dodge the issue that there are categories of mental disturbance with specific courses, and for which we can make specific prognoses, we have no science. Also, there can be no scientific therapy without clinical categories as guidelines to facilitate the study of the life history of specific disturbances, their spontaneous courses, and the interrelationships among causative factors.

The sterility of descriptive and nosological psychiatry occurred when psychoanalysis overpromised answers to questions of etiology through its emphasis on explanation of motivation and meaning. The underemphasis and derogation of clinical observations of behavior were associated with a studied neglect of diagnosis and classification. Such negative approaches have obstructed sound clinical research and, inevitably, studies of casual relations.[5]

Paul Meehl,[6] a distinguished psychologist, makes the important point that, "Rather than decrying nosology, we should become masters of it, recognizing that some of our psychiatric colleagues have in recent times become careless and even unskilled in the art of formal diagnosis."

The problems of organization and the integration of various biological, psychological and social subsystems have occupied much of my own attention. Relevant to this concept, I have focused on anxiety as a system and as a significant variable for a unified theory of human behavior.[7] Until recently, I have been involved in quantities of anxiety, depression and anger as dependent variables that can be estimated with high degrees of reliability, in correlation with other quantitative measures of somatic and social behaviors.

CLASSIFICATIONS

Kraepelin's orginal classifications included hebephrenia, catatonia paranoia, paranoid, schizoaffective, simple, acute undifferentiated, chronic undifferentiated, childhood type and residual schizophrenia. These were based on Koch's postulates for bacterial disease—similar cause, course and outcome—but Kraepelen's "dementia praecox" proved fallacious; the disease was not always associated with dementia and was not always precocious. Eugene Bleuler renamed the condition "schizophrenia," and defined its primary disturbances as the "four A's:" loosening of associations, inappropriate affect, ambivalence and autism.[8]

For decades, the clinical classifications of schizophrenia have followed Kraepelin's original groupings either exactly or, following World War II, with some modifications. Manfred Bleuler,[9/10] who excludes the borderline and the pseudoneurotic diagnoses, classifies schizophrenics in terms of their "long course," using the following patterns:

Straight evolutions

1. Acute onset followed immediately by chronic severe psychosis;

2. Chronic onset leading slowly to chronic severe psychosis;
3. Acute onset followed immediately by chronic mild psychosis;
4. Chronic onset leading slowly to chronic mild psychosis;

Phasic evolutions

5. Several acute episodes leading to chronic severe psychosis;
6. Several acute episodes leading to chronic mild psychosis;
7. One or several acute episodes with outcome in recovery.

Manfred Bleuler's cases, which numbered 208, were followed for 20 years. The diagnosis of schizophrenia was based on disturbed thinking, affective phenomena, depersonalization, delusions and hallucinations. No subject with organic disturbances was included. He included manic and depressive symptoms, if thought disorder was also present, and diagnosed them as schizoaffective. The family life in childhood of each patient was described as "misery." Many who suffered acute psychoses had a long-lasting recovery, while other individuals ended up with severe chronic psychosis—but no special form of treatment was responsible for the outcome one way or the other. Psychological tests, including the Rorschach, did not disclose specific findings for schizophrenia.

In our own researches,[11] we attempt to differentiate acute psychoses, chronic psychoses, paranoid schizophrenic psychoses, schizoaffective schizophrenia and schizophrenia with convulsions. All these classifications are tentative and can only be confirmed by long follow-up studies. Apter[12] adds another subgroup, which he terms "irreversible," to the chronic psychoses.

Going back to my 1953 clinical introduction to Beck's[13] *Six Schizophrenias,* we recognized that the diagnosis of schizophrenia is not easy, certain or quickly achieved. After considerable review of the literature we had to settle on our own definition. In some manner, clinical research on schizophrenia is circular in that patients are so diagnosed (sometimes by experts) and what is found is called a schizophrenic attribute. If what is searched for is not found the condition is not schizophrenic!

In any case, on the basis of the clinical conferences during which our current research team listened to and judged the interviews with patients, our patients were classified into the following diagnostic categories:

1. *Acute schizophrenic psychosis with mixed symptomotology.* This characterized those with sharp, rather suddenly and recently appearing psychotic episodes after a period of previous good adjustment who soon enter into a remission with only little evidence of subsequent disorganization. These individuals can be returned to school or jobs, their families and their social groups.

2. *Chronic schizophrenic psychosis with mixed symptomotology.* This condition indicated long-standing experiences of inner turmoil and social incompetence with clear psychotic symptoms, but without the necessary appearance of an acute psychosis. A gradually developing psychosis is the typical picture.

3. *Paranoid schizophrenic psychosis* designates those who experience frank delusions with a persecutory or grandiose content. They are not typically bizarre in their conventional behavior or even, generally, in their thinking, except when the delusional content is focused on. They also tend to be cautious, suspicious and hyperalert.

4. *Schizophrenic psychosis with convulsions* designates those with generalized seizures preceding an acute schizophrenic

psychotic episode. They do not have jacksonian focal epilepsy, uncinate fits or violent ictal rage attacks.

5. *Schizoaffective psychosis* comprises a group who, in their life histories or during their psychotic attacks, manifest either depressions (as distinguished from anhedonia) or manic behaviors or both, as well as schizophrenic thought disorders. These are quite difficult to diagnose.

6. *Nonschizophrenic* conditions, which include depression monopolar and bipolar, character disorders and neuroses.

At the time of this classificatory interviewing our psychiatrists developed an outline for the accumulation and classification of pertinent data including the past and present. Rorschach data included past tests as well as repeated current tests. Clinical data were available to compare at least two points of time separated by several years, thus giving a fairly adequate estimate of course and outcome. Herewith is the clinical work-outline:

I. *Clinical status*
   A. As evidenced in current behavior elicited by the psychiatric social history.
   B. As determined by the behavior in interview from the verbal and nonverbal productions. The delineation of the clinical picture should be an accurate description of the patient's patterns in work, school, home, etc.; his sexual activities, his attitude towards friends and recreation, his expectations, his concept of self, his attitude toward the past.

I emphasize that the clinical picture as a current segment of the patient's life was described in the terms of the present (this month or this week) time. We were interested in the verbal and nonverbal current behavior, and not influenced by whatever psychotic episode occurred in the past. The most accurate description of the clinical picture was the best way by which we could get an estimation of the ego functions.

II. *Psychodynamic state*
   A. The psychodynamics of the current illness.
   B. The precipitating stimulus to the illness including the meaning of this stimulus to the patient.
   C. The psychodynamics of the premorbid personality (premorbid meaning before any actual overt illness).
   D. The genetic factors, which include both psychological and constitutional, the latter so far as can be estimated.

According to this outline, though, we were then interested in determining what constitutional or developmental factors (genetic) produce a particular type of personality (premorbid) and which stimulus with a particular psychological meaning to the patient acts to precipitate a psychiatric illness.

Our program is *now* oriented toward attempting to define the types, the etiologies and the adaptive meaning of the schizophrenias. The program is open ended in that projects may be added, or even dropped, when indicated. But the basic principle is that a large sample of schizophrenics, constituting a range of symptom pictures, "normal" controls, and other nonschizophrenic psychopathological persons will be available for the same tests over time—including during periods of remission, during clinic or halfway house attendance or when readmitted to a hospital.

The diagnostic data were collected by a semistructured clinical interview conducted with each of the patients. The interview was taped for later listening and assessment of content by a team of clinicians. The interviewer, without prior knowledge of the patient's history or hospital diagnosis (which were obtained at a later date), received each patient in his office after the patient had agreed (by informed consent) to be interviewed and was sufficiently organized and in touch with reality to remain cooperative during the interview. The topics later became the focus for our special rating scales, called the Schizophrenic State Inventory (SSI). We later described and rated the patients' behaviors in the social setting of his nursing unit.

THE MANIFESTATIONS OF SCHIZOPHRENIA

What basic factors are at least knowable about schizophrenic people? The questions encompass biogenetic, epidemiological, familial, psychological, biochemical and sociological evidence.* Surely, a behavioral outcome like schizophrenia cannot be explained by a single causal entity. Indeed, the bewildering array of symptom pictures argues against a research strategy that searches for a single etiological factor. The complexity of schizophrenic phenomena, the changing manifestations of the process within a single person, the vast individual differences in appearance and course and the influence of social factors on the course of the process all speak for strategies of study that reflect a confrontation with a system of interrelated and mutually transacting components.

Macfie Campbell[14] wrote in 1935:

> Instead of considering patients with the diagnosis dementia praecox as having a "disease," I prefer to think of them as belonging to a Greek letter society, the conditions for admission to which are obscure; inclusion in and exclusion from the fraternity are determined by considerations which may vary from year to

*Parts of this section are taken from Grinker, R. R. Sr., and Holzman, P. S. Schizophrenic pathology in young adults. *Archives of General Psychiatry,* 1973, **28;** 168–175. (© 1973 by the American Medical Association.)

year and from place to place, and the directing board is not known.

We must develop a new research strategy when we further consider that the forms of the schizophrenias we are most familiar with—the hospitalized patients in acute or chronic phase with or without paranoid symptoms—are not the only variations of the schizophrenias, nor, it appears, are they the most frequent ones. Nonpsychotic forms of schizophrenia (for example, ambulatory and latent schizophrenia, as well as schizoid character) may claim a wider prevalence than do the familiar psychotic forms.

One must now take very seriously the *protean manifestations* of schizophrenia. To restrict research on schizophrenia to the classic acute and chronic psychotic forms of the disorder—that is, people whose dislocations are so severe that they must be hospitalized—may force our attention to dysfunction which is correlated with severity or with deterioration, and away from the essence of the schizophrenic syndrome. For we now realize that social deterioration is a secondary and not inevitable, accompaniment to the schizophrenic syndrome. Focusing on social and personal functioning confuses what is intrinsic with what may be a consequence of schizophrenia.

For these reasons, the research enterprise we have undertaken focuses on a range of schizophrenias. The studies, in cooperation and collaboration with a number of investigators, are a loose federation, guided only by the theoretical orientation that emphasizes the systems approach, and by the multiple and overlapping studies on the same groups of patients. We describe one group of patients not usually studied in research on schizophrenia: young adults from middle and upper socioeconomic groups, hospitalized for what appeared to be acute psychotic episodes. Although each of these patients has been studied by a number of tests, including psychological, psychomotor, vestibular, memory, perceptual, family interaction, cognitive controls and biochemical, we will describe here only the psychological characteristics of this special group of patients exposed during interviews.

However, before getting down to specifics, let us quote an abstract of Jones's[15] critical review of methods for studying the development of schizophrenia: a review that has been very valuable in our work:

The assets and liabilities of current methodologies for studying the development of schizophrenia are reviewed under three major headings: retrospective methods which draw inferences concerning developmental factors in the lives of subjects who are already ill by using data collected after the onset of the illness, childhood records which draw developmental inferences about pathology in adults on the basis of developmental data contained in records collected previously during childhood, and prospective or "high risk" methods which examine developmental factors in subjects not yet ill but having a higher than normal probabilitiy of becoming ill. The primary focus of the review is upon the relative capacities of existing methodologies to generate developmental statements at a high degree of specificity and validity. Retrospective methods reviewed include the systematic use of the case history interview, direct observations of patients' behavior, psychological testing, and family interaction experiments. Childhood records examined include both "follow-back" methods in which early life events of adult patients are collected from childhood records and also "follow-up" methods in which a sample of subjects for whom childhood records are available is followed up in adulthood. Prospective methods examined include experimental designs employing a variety of strategies (longitudinal, cross-sectional, and compound designs) and criteria for selecting a high risk population. The advantages of prospective methods in solving methodological roadblocks inherent in retrospective and childhood records are discussed along with their liabilities.

The constantly changing "what" of schizophrenia is at present characterized by disorders of thinking, feelings, perception and motor functions. We emphasize here that when we use the term schizophrenia we do not necessarily mean psychosis, which is a behavioral term, applicable as well to other conditions such as toxicities, infections, traumas and organic brain syndromes. We include in the schizophrenic syndrome the nonpsychotic manifestations of the schizophrenias—that is, the so-called latent, pre-, incipient, ambulatory and remitted schizophrenics, as well as those who have what has been called schizophrenic characters.

Thought disorders. It has long been considered that thought disorders constitute a primary and pathognomic* indication of schizophrenia. Harrow[16/17] and his group at Yale University have studied thought disorders carefully through a wide variety of psychological tests, with confusing results. They conclude that thought disorders are probably primary in acute schizophrenics but question their presence in remissions. Harrow is continuing this research at our Institute. Idiosyncratic thinking occurs in chronic schizophrenics; personalized thinking in both acute and nonschizophrenic psychoses.

We have attempted to define sharply the thought disorder, including conceptual overinclusions. These seem to decrease in remissions, but further research needs to be done on whether disordered thinking persists after an acute breakdown. Studies of differential response to drugs, premorbid and morbid signs and symptoms have usually failed as predictors of outcome.[16/17/18] Overinclusion,

---

*Pathognomic designates any sign or symptom whose presence makes the diagnosis certain.

which indicates defects in attention and perception, is associated with anxiety and is found in all acute psychotics. In schizophrenia, disordered thinking appears clearest in complex unstructured situations revealing no specific content. Chronic schizophrenics have more concrete thinking, and the young intellectual schizophrenic seems to have less deficit in social competence. Each of the above statements could be disputed by other investigators conducting equally good research. In conclusion, thought disorder on which experienced clinicians base their diagnosis of schizophrenia must be included.

In mild cases of schizophrenic psychoses and even in nonpsychotic schizophrenics, the thought disorder may be mild, sporadic or occasional, and may, in its very mildness, tend to be overlooked in ordinary conversation, simply because one can fill in the communicational gaps. Yet, in careful listening to tape recordings of schizophrenic patients, the thought "slippage" can be discerned. For example, the patient may omit ideas essential to the listener's grasp of continuity (ellipsis), as if the patient assumed that the listener must know the full thoughts. Occasionally, even in mild cases, words will be used idiosyncratically, or idiosyncratic words will be used (neologisms). For example, the word "barbituary" was used by a patient to describe his attempt to commit suicide by ingesting barbiturates; a highly intelligent young patient described his recent arrest by the police, and called the charge against him a "misendeamor." Inquiry into these words and into ellipsis generally brings out some thought confusion, fluid ideas and even delusions.

In more severely disorganized patients, the kinds of thought disorder variously described by many investigators are extant, such as autistic intrusions, predicative thinking, blocking, flooding, incoherence, concreteness, neophobia, overinclusiveness and paralogical thinking. These aspects of schizophrenic thinking can be observed either under resting or stress conditions. That their incidence increases under stress implicates stress only as a potentiator and not as a cause of the slippage. Further, these instances of thought disorder are observed when the patient shows a clear sensorium and is not necessarily fatigued, toxic or otherwise in an altered state of consciousness. Although some gifted people can approximate such instances of slippage, as in humor or in poetic or theoretic literary devices, these artistic people are deliberately striving for these effects. With schizophrenic patients, however, they are not produced for artistic effects and they are not under voluntary control.

Thought disorders may be apparent in one or several psychological acts, such as perceiving, speaking, recalling, writing. Most schizophrenic patients manifest thought disorder in the course of communicative behavior. Our view is that the presence of thought disorders does not necessarily implicate a specific defect of the part process in which it is seen—e.g., language, behavior, perception, memory, attention. Rather, it may reflect a more general impairment or dysfunction in the capacity to organize sensory and ideational experiences or to maintain the organization of ideas and percepts which had once been established.

Other Characteristics of Schizophrenia. A study of all our patients strongly suggests that a pervasive difficulty in maintaining *organizational coherence* is characteristic of all schizophrenics, regardless of type. In the acute phases of the disorder, patients struggle to keep from being flooded by sensory stimulation. Moreover, even beyond the acute phase of the psychosis, the texture of meaning and organization that has the coherence of nonschizophrenic persons seems to be weakened. During periods of remission some patients state, "I feel that I have better control but the difficulties I experienced are still there but in lesser degree." Percepts and ideas are organized in a fluid manner and both the external world and self-feelings are marked by instability. During the early phases of the illness, patients struggle desperately to keep order in their thoughts, affects, actions and perception. Yet, in periods of remission or in nonpsychotic schizophrenic periods, the quality of organizational instability is also prominent.

A second feature of all schizophrenics in our groups of patients is their *pleasureless demeanor*. Although some schizophrenic patients have reported having had fun during childhood, for the most part these young patients report a pervasive inability to derive much joy from life. Even when moderately successful in their accomplishments during their hospitalization, they showed a kind of dampening in their joy and an absence of pleasure. This agrees rather strikingly with Rado's impression that anhedonia is a crucial symptom, not only of schizophrenia, but of schizotypic persons. He believed that, with a proprioceptive diathesis and inherited or acquired anxiety, the *integrating* power of pleasure is deficient. In contrast, the nonschizophrenic hospitalized patients could describe episodes of enjoyment, not only in retrospect, but even in their present hospitalization. Further, the view of their own future described by the schizophrenic patients held little prospect of amelioration.

A third feature of the schizophrenic group as a whole was the predominance of *excessive dependency*. This tendency is obvious not only in the relationships of patients to their families, but also as patients to the hospital, staff and particularly to their therapists. Examples of this dependency include relapses when a patient's therapist is away on vacation and when nurses leave or are shifted to another unit. In the interviews, patients spontaneously and clearly indicate their need to maintain a dependency relationship. In answer to a specific question: "What would happen if your mother died?" Patients frequently respond with a variety of tragic answers: "I'd go to pieces;" "I would fall apart;" "I couldn't live;" "I would go crazy again;" "I would be too scared to continue."

A fourth noteworthy feature of these patients is the unmistakable *deficiency in competence*. Although the patients in our schizophrenic groups are all within the normal-to-superior range of intelligence, they were achieving less than one would have expected by virtue of their intellectual endowment. These instances of incompetence included poor school performance, poor job performance and accepting jobs that were clearly below their capabilities. Although the most clearly incompetent patients were those in the chronic schizophrenic group, none of the patients in the other schizophrenic groups could be considered to be competent. At the conclusion of their hospitalization, most of the schizophrenics accept this fact and lower their goals for future careers.

A fifth feature is *the precipitant* for the hospitalization. In most, but not all, schizophrenic patients the precipitating event of the psychosis or of the hospitalization was a challenge to their self-esteem. For some patients it was the breakup of a love relationship; for others, it was leaving home for the first time to enter college (a situation that makes claims as well on the excessive dependency of these patients); and for still others, it was a rebuff of a person important to them, such as a teacher, an employer or a doctor.

As for the age of onset of the psychosis, only in the chronic group could we find evidence for clear psychotic behavior in childhood. Other patients seemed to be free of psychosis until the episode that brought them to the hospital in their late teens or early 20s. However, there were indications in all patients of their excessive dependency, degree of anhedonia, diminished competence, and pervasive difficulty in feeling themselves as cohesive and integrated persons with a continuity in time and with an enduring organization. This feeling of *fragmentation* was strikingly exaggerated during the psychotic periods. For example, one patient ("acute schizophrenia"), when looking into the mirror, believed that she was becoming her mother. This feeling of fragmentation is accompanied by an overwhelming feeling of anxiety which most of the time has the content of "going to pieces," or of "going crazy." These periods of overwhelming anxiety generally forced the patients to remain isolated, either in their rooms or off in lonely places, playing the guitar, listening to a radio, or simply daydreaming. Although the acute experiences of fragmentation diminished with treatment, and when the acute phase of the illness ebbed, the fragmentation seemed to be a quasi-permanent low-level concern of these patients throughout their lives. They frequently report, "I never really felt that I knew who I was," or "I was doing what I thought my father wanted me to, but I really don't know what I wanted to do."

It was striking that these young schizophrenic patients were able to maintain appropriate behavior during the interview, despite periods of psychotic and highly variable behavior on the nursing unit. This seems to indicate that some parts of the self-system operate on a more mature level despite the lack of development and/or regression of other parts.

Pending the outcome of a number of focused laboratory studies, we believe that the following *qualities* distinguish the young schizophrenic patients from those who are not so diagnosed: (1) the presence of a disorder of thinking, even though it is subtly present; (2) a striking quality of diminished capacity to experience pleasure, particularly in interpersonal relationships; (3) a strong characterological dependency upon people; (4) a noteworthy impairment in competence; (5) an exquisitely vulnerable sense of self-regard.

We would suppose that these five qualities reflect a more

basic, hypothetical dysfunction in maintaining the kind of organization necessary for appropriate, adaptive orientation to one's surroundings and to oneself. This basic disorder, we would further hypothesize, need not lead inevitably to psychosis. The loose adherence to stable organizations may sometimes lead to reorganizations of reality that may even have social, artistic, or scientific value. We would suppose, however, that a significant degree of competence among other factors would be necessary for such an outcome.

THE "HOW:" BIOLOGY, PSYCHOLOGY, SOCIOLOGY

We have attempted to approach the problem of the schizoprenias on the tentative assumption that it is a *heterogeneous syndrome.* This has meant that we have tried to cover, at least in part, the tremendous literature in books, periodicals, abstracts and summaries. Complete coverage was obviously impossible because genetic, constitutional, biochemical and physical dysfunction, anomalies of development (both physiological and psychological), interpersonal experiences, anxiety and regression all had to be included. Likewise, the psychological and sociological frames of reference and the peer groups of infancy, childhood, adolescence, young adulthood and adulthood must be included.

The problems of organization and the integration of various sub-systems; biological, psychological, and social have occupied much of my own attention. We assume that the disturbed behaviors and the aberrant thinking, the affective and motor functions constitute phenomena overlaying processes that are concealed from direct observation, description and measurement. If we liken these phenomena to the projections of an iceberg above the surface of the sea, clues may be obtained regarding the hidden or submerged structures.

Many investigators in this field, beginning with Bleuler, have been concerned with attempts to differentiate primary from secondary characteristics of schizophrenia and to distinguish "defenses" (for example, obsessions, hypochondriasis and a facade of normality) from that which is primary. Despite the great variability among schizophrenics and, from time to time, within each individual, clinical experience indicates that a basic and terrifying anxiety is primary. In my opinion, this anxiety may not be only quantitatively great, but it may have a *special quality*.

A special quality of anxiety in the process of development may influence the organization of the symbolic internal world in the direction of constant or variable preparation for danger. This in turn could influence the subject's interpretation of his external world and determine the defective organization and control of his symbolic thinking.

Relevant to this concept, I have focused on anxiety as a system and as a significant variable for a unified theory of human behavior.[7] Until recently I have been involved in quantities of anxiety, depression and anger as dependent variables which can be estimated with high degrees of reliability, in correlation with other quantitative measures of somatic and social behaviors.

As the determinant of a system, anxiety* denotes processes or organization involving total behavior in the social environment, cognitive and perceptive functioning, and physiological actions, all of which are adaptive under conditions in which anxiety exists, often outlasting the consciously reportable affect. The total system is involved with

*A portion of this discussion on anxiety is taken from: Grinker, R. R. Sr. Anxiety as a significant variable for a unified theory of human behavior. *Archives of General Psychiatry* 1959 (© 1959 by the American Medical Association), 1: 537–556.

the environment in that external conditions or internal dis
turbances acting on the anxiety system may augment its
component activities; or stimulate the total organism to
remove itself to safety from the dangerous stimulus to
which it is highly sensitive; or may stimulate an attack, in
attempting to destroy the danger. Thus, even if interest is
focused on anxiety as an organization, with its multiplicity
of component parts, transactions that involve environmental parameters are ever present. The total social and interpersonal setting in which the subject lives and moves
should, therefore, be taken into account, either by observing its changes or by controlling its constancy as much as
possible.

Anxiety may be categorized quantitatively as either
facilitative or destructive of psychological functions; i.e., it
can result in alertness, preparatory apprehension-"free,"
or panic. The terms signal and traumatic anxiety, of psychoanalytic theory can be classified in the same way. In fact,
our entire psychiatric nosological classification is based on
techniques utilized by man to avoid or minimize the un-
bearable feeling of impending doom when anxiety is
"free."

Signal anxiety which is evoked by a foreboding of danger, is related to ego strengths and sensitivities which are
partly constitutional and partly experiential (learned).
Much has been learned about the factors that influence
psychological conditioning in early life, and that prepare
the subject to cope adequately with a changing environment. Sufficient feeding, proper temperature regulations,
adequate sensory stimulation and body contact, contrast
with many items indicating inadequate care when the infant
is dependent on external controls. Identification with current cultural patterns through incorporation of value systems is necessary for adequate social existence. All of these
—proper nutrition, stimulation, ideals, prohibitions and
value systems—seem to be incorporated and effective for

preparation against later strains if administered in proper doses at the right times.

If, however, these early evidences of stability are not present anxiety is the likely result. Unfortunately, early in life, defensive aggression or withdrawal may mask the affect. Secondary symptoms such as withdrawal and dereistic unrealistic thinking may be protective defenses against actualization of danger in reality. Therefore the quantity and quality of anxiety may be masked until exposed by catastrophic experiences or by uncovering procedures. It is then that the anxiety is revealed to be related to the expectation of destruction of the self with dissolution of already weak ego boundaries and loss of identity.

Although the quantities of anxiety or, for that matter, any affect may be estimated, qualities require descriptions by the subject or/and inferences by an observer. A major difficulty is, of course, the natural human tendency to explain or rationalize undesirable feelings on the basis of external events. *Neurotic anxiety* as we see it in our patients, experienced as a feeling of impending doom, is usually focal in relation to some event and is time-limited. *Anxiety in schizophrenics* is a horrible generalized fear of dissolution and loss of personal control. It is more like a survival threat.

The functional predisposition or proneness to anxiety of an individual is reflected in his current psychodynamics, the genesis of which is rather complicated. Persons laden with irrational guilt feelings are more easily stimulated to anticipate harm to themselves. Those who have a great deal of shame are often made anxious by situations that include the possibility of failure. The most effective and generally *universal* stimulation for anxiety is isolation, and/or absence or distortion of communications leading to a feeling of impending disintegration. In the somatic sphere, there are similar general predispositions, such as change of temperature, especially cold, physical trauma, bleeding and fatigue. Individual predispositions are not, as in the psychological system, subject to categorization, but are referable to early somatic conditioning; this conditioning, if known, could possibly form the basis of prediction of intensity and duration of stress responses to a particular stimulus. In the social field, situations contributing to the feeling of not belonging or not conforming, as indicated by attitudes of those around, evoke severe psychological reactions of anxiety, as well as retreat of the individual toward more isolation or to an attack on the environment.

The above statements indicate clearly, I believe, that anxiety is a response which may be activated by meaningful cues that suggest danger to the person, and that it initiates preparatory activities. When these fail, psychological disintegration may result. Signal anxiety is a sensitive indicator, an alarm.

What we term the resting or idling state is not quiescent. Although relatively silent, it is characterized by well-patterned structural processes of adaptation within a relatively stable homeostatic internal environment. When this is disturbed, appropriate local systems become activated, bearing the brunt of adjustment, although with repercussions throughout the organism. One or more systems may bear the essential brunt of disequilibrium, avoiding a greater spread of disturbance. With more intense stimuli, or when the stimuli last longer, more and more systems are activated into heightened responses, including central nervous system participation. It is in the later phases that the entire orchestra of visceral activity becomes activated into synchronous, rather than out-of-phase, responses.

A priori we are not able to indicate the relationship between a quality of anxiety and disturbances of the central nervous system as expressed in cognitive dysfunctions, not necessarily in linear or causal sequences. No matter whether the antecedent known variable is a quality of anxiety or a central nervous system defect, endocrine imbalance or traumatic experiences in infancy, the expression of the defect will be in the psychological experience of, or defense against, *loss of control.* Holzman's[19] theory of feedback deficit in persons with high levels of arousal postulates the search for massive stimuli in order for stimulation to be effective in shutting off the patient's response.

Epstein and Coleman,[20] as we have quoted in Chapter XII, believe that schizophrenics have a heightened drive arousal associated with a low threshold for disorganization with resulting stimulus overgeneralization. On the other hand, chronic schizophrenics have developed reduced drive quantities. Narrowed attention is protective in that it reduces the quantity of input down to a level the schizophrenic can handle.

Why does the schizophrenic adaptation often take the form of increasing simplification of psychic activities and a move toward less complexity? The excited disruptions of behavior or mentation in the acute schizophrenic may represent the disturbance-in-process. Eventually the adaptation called schizophrenia becomes effective and chronic, and the subject arrives at a more quiescent phase of regression and withdrawal. It is not known whether the lack of a more healthy adaptation is due to the overwhelming character of anxiety, the innate absence of coping behaviors, the lack of learned methods of coping or an organizational defect.

The task of determining the validity of the hypothesis that anxiety is qualitatively different in schizophrenia is difficult. It cannot be determined in a quiescent state, but requires a challenge to the organization. This requires the tasks of observing spontaneous challenges in life situations, imposing verbal challenges or distorting communication, or utilizing anxiety-producing drugs such as epinephrine. Then we may obtain introspective accounts from the subject, observe behaviors such as withdrawal, new or increased psychotic behavior, attacks on the object from which the stress stimulus emerges, etc. Since we are interested in quality and not quantity, measurements are not important at this time. Rather we are interested in trends toward changes in behaviors that can be observed and described.

The most meticulously carried out quantitative surveys on isolated functions do not demonstrate significant variables in the schizophrenia system. We demonstrated the same results in our work on psychosomatic disturbances of combat neuroses. A demonstrable quality of disturbed function needs first to be isolated from the vast array of psychological phenomena in order subsequently to investigate its basic underlying elements.

I believe that the times are propitious for the abandonment of overall surveys in favor of investigations derived from specified theoretical propositions, whether these start with a study of genes, infantile experiences, family constellations, forms of communication, anxiety systems or cognitive functions, not as ends themselves. In order to understand the system we call schizophrenia, we need to be more certain that we know its parts, among which is anxiety and its organizing weakness.*

Not only do most clinical researches utilize a one-shot cross-sectional study, but many utilize only a small number of subjects, thereby increasing variability. Variations in chronicity of the disease, the age and intelligence of the subjects, the situation in which they are studied, the clinical experience of the investigators, the imposed stress, etc. influence the results. Most important are two significant problems. One is the *universal* shifting symptomatology of the clinical syndromes from dramatic overt behavior to quieter, constricted characteristics. The second is the shift in the *individual* disturbance. The schizophrenic in an acute breakdown often reveals all the previously described and

---

*In this chapter, oriented toward the goal of the need for integration of parts of the schizophrenic system, some brief repetition of what has appeared in previous chapters is necessary.

classical symptoms, as well as the premorbid flooding of thoughts, confusion, anxiety, hallucinations and paranoia.[21] The schizophrenic in a remission is often superficially indistinguishable from a healthy person.

We need to bear in mind that there are profound differences between the essence of diseases like schizophrenia, the challenges that bring out their overt forms, the subsequent regressions and the possible adaptations. Grinker and Holzman[11] state:

> Sufficient evidence is available to determine that the dysfunctions in the schizophrenias implicate biological (for example, biogenetic), psychological (for example, childhood experiences), and environmental (for example, stressors) realms. We assume that life challenges ranging from serious illnesses or structural anomalies in infancy to narcissistic injuries are necessary to precipitate a predisposed (schizotaxic) individual into a psychosis, given the proper environmental field.

As Holzman[19] states:

> The schizophrenic syndrome is a process, with varied and protean pictures. It may develop in early or late childhood or in early or late adulthood; it may develop insidiously with no acute psychotic disruption or it may erupt suddenly and unexpectedly; it may never recur or it may never go on to recovery, or it may re-occur once or many times, each time with a poorer remission. The symptoms may be mild or serious. The premorbid pictures may range widely, too. A theory that takes account of only one manifestation of schizophrenic illness—such as the loss of effective reality testing, for example—can only be an *ad hoc* and incomplete theory. The complexity of the phenomena make it no longer possible to ignore the systems aspect of the schizophrenias.

A systems approach can envelop the broad sweep of schizophrenic phenomena. Whether one chooses to study etiological factors—genic, biochemical, familial, demographic—or the responses to such factors—including the inner resources of the person—depends upon one's proclivities and interests. But we should not mistake any of these aspects of the pathology for the complete picture of disease or of *the* treatment. It is the imbalance among all these factors—between internal and external threats and pressures on the one hand, and the organism's efforts to maintain itself by thoughts, feelings, somatic shifts, and changed social relationships—that may be called the disease.

BIOLOGICAL COMPONENTS OF SCHIZOPHRENIA

Despite the current antipsychiatric contention that schizophrenia is a nondisease and only a label psychiatrists have devised to give them power over the public, the majority of investigators believe that *a strong biological component* constitutes part of the etiological matrix of this disorder. In Chapter VIII, the monozygotic twin studies of Kallman[22] and Rosenthal,[23] including Rosenthal and Kety's critique[24] indicating that heredity has been overemphasized in the etiology of schizophrenia, have been mentioned and need not be repeated.

Kringlen,[25] on the other hand, indicates two questions are asked in genetics: *"What* is inherited? *How* is it inherited? "The first question may be answered by twin studies, the second by genealogical studies which should be extended past the period of risk. He states:

> In the investigations so far, this pattern seems consistent: The more accurate and careful the samplings, the lower the concordance figures. In the present study of an unselected sample of 342 pairs of twins, 35 to 64 years of age, where one or both at some time in their

lives had been hospitalized for a "functional psychosis", the concordance figures for schizophrenia were
found to be 25 to 38 percent in monozygotics and 4
to 10 percent in dizygotics. These concordance rates
support a genetic factor in the etiology of schizophrenia; however, the genetic factor does not play as great
a role as has been assumed. As more research in this
area has progressed, monozygotic twins have been
found to be more discordant than concordant for
schizophrenia.

Another approach to the biogenesis of schizophrenia involves the study of adult schizophrenics between 20 and 40
years of age who were adopted in childhood. Their biological parents were more likely to be mentally ill than their
adopted parents, whose good parenting could not overcome the biological potential. In general, parents and siblings of schizophrenic patients had a high morbidity rate.
But higher morbidity of what? It seems quite certain, based
both on years of clinical experience by practicing psychiatrists and on recent experimental investigations, that families of schizophrenics contain more members with some
form of mental illness than members with adequate controls. Yet, to call all these forms of deviation parts of a
"schizophrenic spectrum" serves only to confuse for the
sake of maintaining theoretical constructs.[26]
Even the most reductionistic geneticists state that symptoms are not inherited but are developed by environmental
social factors acting on genetic predispositions.[27] Most are
convinced of the polygenetic theory, not simple Mendelian
inheritance, and the diathesis-stress model. On the other
hand, we should not be content to state that for schizophrenia there are no morbid genes or specific psychological
stresses, and speak only of unfavorable family conditions.[28]
True, there are hidden schizophrenics whose private lives
are filled with magic, mysticism and day dreams, and some
may even be creative.[10]

Other early biological predispositions include varieties of damage to the brain. Among these are intrauterine disturbances in circulation, infections, toxins, birth injuries, neonatal infections, trauma, etc. These are said to be evidenced by "soft" neurological signs in the infant.[29] Unfortunately, by the time subjects have reached adolescence or adulthood these are mostly invisible because of compensations and they cannot be diagnosed with any degree of certainty.

In the current era of psychopharmacology, numerous studies have indicated some biochemical abnormalities in schizophrenic patients. Unfortunately, a wide variety of metabolic errors have been described. Probably the most universally accepted general concept is a disturbance in transmethylization affecting central nervous system catechole-amine metabolism due to an overactivity of dopamine. Aside from this deficiency concept, there are theories with challengeable experiments that schizophrenia is caused by an autoimmune disorder,[30] a vitamin deficiency and a plasma protein factor[31] that alters the lactate-pyruvic acid ratio in chicken erythrocytes. Also, in monozygotic twins discordant for schizophrenia, the nondialyzed platelets of the schizophrenic twin had much higher levels of enzyme ability to form the hallucinogen dimethyltryptamine.

Where the abnormal biochemical activity resides in the brain is not known, but the hypothalamus seems to be the appropriate target. It is interesting that Schildkraut and Kety[27] state that the biochemical abnormalities do not indicate genetic or constitutional causes, but may be due to early environmental factors.

A number of other biological studies include disturbances of sleep rhythm involving a reduction of stage four and reduction of total time of sleep. The average evoked potential is reported to be in abnormally narrower ranges.[32] Patients with periodic catatonia are said to have a thyroid deficiency. Many EEG studies have produced a variety of unconfirmed results, but modern fine-grained studies used in our laboratory by Giannitrapani and Kayton[33] show:

> The findings indicate that EEG autospectra show correlates to a portion of the patients having the primary diagnosis of schizophrenia in this study. Even though these findings await confirmation, the manner in which the scores in the 19 and 29 Hz band are distributed for the schizophrenics points to the possibility that spectrum analysis of the EEG could ultimately prove useful in differentiating between the disorders which are currently subsumed under the general heading of schizophrenia.

Heath,[30] using electrodes inserted in the midline paraventricular areas of humans reports abnormal spikes in schizophrenics. Grinker and Serota,[34/35] using both hypothalamic and surface leads showed that schizophrenics, in contrast to "normal" persons, evinced little electrical reaction to cold, intravenous adrenaline, verbal stimuli, and that electrical stimulation through the hypothalamic lead produced little cortical response. Intravenous injection of sodium amytal evoked both hypothalamic and cortical responses.

Holzman, Procter and Hughes[36] report studies of eye movements following the swing of a pendulum:

> Smooth pursuit eye movements, reflecting as they do the coordination of eye velocity with object velocity, represent a critical factor in visual perception. Their impairment in schizophrenic patients may be associated with the impaired and idiosyncratic reality appraisal typical of these patients, for visual perception, a central factor in reality contact, involves the organization of the entire perceptual system and requires effective motor response and feedback for its adaptive task.

Finally, we come to a generalization not only based on many direct tests of autonomic functions but also used on clinical observations focused on anxiety, perception, cognition etc. that schizophrenics suffer from autonomic over-excitement and vigilance. They attempt to defend themselves against this quality but they seem unable to habituate themselves to exciting stimuli.

PSYCHOLOGICAL COMPONENTS OF SCHIZOPHRENIA

Modern *psychological research* has been effective in moving our interest in diagnosis from the primary and secondary symptoms of schizophrenia to more sophisticated approaches. To name a few studies, Holzman[19] focuses on a defect in perceptual feedback; Spohn[37] finds a deficiency in information processes because of inconstant attention; Burnham[38] has studied inadequate differentiation and integration leading to faulty object relations, lack of autonomy and unreliable reality constructs; Shakow[39] discusses neophobia, lack of spontaneity, faculty scanning and articulation, etc. It is interesting that most of these investigators attempt to articulate their interpretations with biological, especially autonomic, failures. *It may be generalized that weak central control and organizational abnormalities should be closely related to pervasive qualitatively deficient homeostatic regulation.*
What we as psychologists and psychiatrists study are the psychological and behavioral emergent manifestations of primary, *i.e.* basic, biological defects. From these emergent phenomena, clues may be obtained that point to variables in the schizophrenic concept and its subcategories. Basically this is a systems approach from which concepts of the schizophrenias may be improved beyond the simple-minded diagnoses for clinical purposes.[40]
A recent major concept of the genesis of schizophrenia concerns *the family* as a system of communications. Are these distorted communications causal to or as a result of

a single schizophrenic member of a family? We may consider communications as quantitatively too much or too little, and qualitatively distorted or indicating overprotectiveness or overcontrol.[3] Experienced clinicians have long recognized that in treating schizophrenic patients they are often blocked by interference from one or both disturbed parents.

Mishler and Waxler[41] have reviewed the current theories of family interaction processes and schizophrenia. Bateson's "double bind" conceives of incongruent negative injunctions. Lidz[42] writes about a distorted or fragmented developmental milieu based on psychoanalytic theory. The mothers of ill daughters are poorly organized, leading to "schizmatic" results. The fathers of sons are weak and present no model, leading to "skewed" relationships. Wynne[43] found that families of schizophrenics were not stable and that a facade of pseudomutuality is common. This is a model based on role relations.

There is a great interest in the family of origin of schizophrenics.* Methods of study vary: interviewing all members, using psychological tests on all members singly and together and observing and hearing the family as its members perform tasks together. This area of research is important, but as yet various investigators have published discordant findings.[44]

---

* *Childhood autism* is a peculiar puzzle seemingly not the same as schizophrenia. The early investigators considered autism as a developmental product of cold overintellectual parents—a psychogenic theory. More research showed that parents of these children were not guilty as reported. On the other hand, the learning patterns (lack of capacity to transfer information from one sensory system to another—cross + modal learning), low intelligence, EEG's, poor memory, all suggest central nervous system damage to hypothalamic or limbic lobe functions.[45] Despite reports of improvement in autistic children by increased body contact to improve the body ego, operant conditioning, drug administration, etc. the acceptable major evidence is that childhood autism is an incurable organic defect of the central nervous system. Yet there are suggestions that infantile autism, childhood schizophrenia and adult schizophrenia represent failures of integration of cognitive and perceptual systems and that each represents a different developmental level at which such integration fails.

However, the early studies of childhood schizophrenics by Bender[46] revealed disturbances in mobility, perception and emotional responses. These children tend to "melt" into available adults, have a maturational lag and developmental unevenness. Her predictions, from these phenomena and tonelessness after twirling the children, that they would become schizophrenics were validated after 20 years of follow-up.

Escalona and Heider[47] could predict future neurotic disturbances by observing infants in their natural settings. Brody[48] likewise laid the ground work for studies of infants by observing them in transactions with their mothers during feeding, changing diapers, fondling and letting them alone, from which predictions could be made. Gesell and Amatruda[49] observed respiratory patterns, sleeping, waking, muscle tone and tonic neck reflexes to predict future neuropsychiatric abnormalities.

Studies of "high-risk" children from schizophrenic parents (one or both) has not resulted in definitive conclusions.[50/51] They seemed to reveal behavioral difficulties, but that they too developed schizophrenia cannot be affirmed.[52]

Shakow[53] has studied the schizophrenias for many years within a multidisciplinary group. He has developed hypotheses based on continuous and difficult empirical studies. In his view, the schizophrenic patient has an aversion to the new (neophobia), and clings to what he has known and done before. Reaction time is slower than with normals and is affected by interpolated stimuli. He hangs on to the old and fails to habituate. Shakow's *set theory* indicates that the schizophrenic cannot maintain a "major set" or readiness to respond to a coming stimulus. He is easily distracted by chance stimuli from the inner or outer environment. He establishes minor sets because of his overwhelming anxiety. In other words, because of his need for love and security he partially regresses, but does maintain islands of integrity. Koh, Kayton and Berry[54] have found that short-term memory is deficient in schizophrenia.

Also, Koh and Kayton[55] in our laboratory studied the recall performance of young nonpsychotic schizophrenics. They report as follows:

> The recall performance of the young non-psychotic schizophrenics is inferior to that of the normals even when the experimenter has minimized introduction of contextual constrains into the recall task; and that this recall deficit of the schizophrenics is, at least in part, attributable to a combined operation of their limited primary and secondary memory capacities, inefficiency in utilizing the stimulus contiguity for mnemonic organization, vulnerability to intrusions and slow response time.

Psychoanalysis as a part of psychology has contributed greatly to the theory of psychiatry, especially since Freud unknowingly attempted to analyse schizophrenias, thereby getting in touch early and quickly with primary process thinking. But schizophrenia and neuroses do not form a continuum and schizophrenia is not explained by psychoanalytic metapsychology or conflict theory. Rather, according to Holzman,[19] there is poor control of the perception-cognitive processing, not only in the patient, but in members of his family. Proprioception and autonomic adjustment are not effected by proper perceptive feed-back.

Dunham,[56] one of the pioneers investigating urban areas with high schizophrenic populations, has recently reviewed *socio-cultural* studies of schizophrenia. As with other investigations, this research is handicapped by the lack of hard criteria for the diagnosis of schizophrenia. Dunham divides the diagnoses into the "soft" and "hard." His studies of schizophrenics in "skidrow" areas created a controversy between the social effects of the area and the *drift* of schizo-phrenics *into* those areas.

Demographic studies regarding the race, sex linkage, or socio-economic classes most susceptible to schizophrenia are not convincing, although lower-class patients are more likely to be chronic. Crosscultural investigations have also not been definitive. One questions: "What is culture-free and culture-fair?"

Lin Yi-Chiang[57] has developed a *theory of role-identity* con-fusion in schizophrenia. There is a protracted struggle be-tween receptivity and responsibility dramatized by its effect on self-identity:

> Findings on the schizophrenic person's major strains center on the ways in which social role expectations and value orientation of the culture or sub-culture affect his self-esteem and self-identity. But role-expec-tations and value orientations are not wholly responsi-ble for the schizophrenic person's protracted unresolved dilemma between dependence and inde-pendence-responsibility. It should be pointed out here that we cannot ignore the schizophrenic person's own participation in the process of creating this role dilemma, the origin of which can be traced back to childhood socialization processes in family interac-tions.

DEVELOPING A UNIFIED APPROACH

Now the big question is, how do we integrate this infor-mation?

The disciplines, methods and languages we have dis-cussed are widely separated. Of course, we can talk about overarching theories such as general systems theory, uni-fied theory or communications[58/59/60] theory. A study of the literature concerned with schizophrenia reveals repetitive statements of theory and of empirical observations whose relevance is obscure, producing, in fact, many "little answers" that are difficult to integrate.[5]

To review the psychological literature on schizophrenia could not only be an herculean, but an impossible task. Thousands of tests are applied to small numbers of patients without knowing really what the test tests. Hardly any are validated or replicated, but the journals are full of them. They have not advanced our knowledge by much. Holley and Nilsson[61] consider that failure to demonstrate validities of clinical tests may be attributed, not to the tests, but to the validation procedure utilized.

The student soon arrives at a point of redundancy of information or "noise." The levels of complexity are so many that theories emphasizing simplicity and parsimony are too limited and those emphasizing generalities are too global. What we call theories are collections of related propositions, not "facts." Unfortunately, as yet, "facts" or empirical observations on schizophrenia lack adequate precision and definition.

The problems associated with schizophrenia demonstrate clearly that there is no single cause and that *multiple factors* enter into every aspect of cause, course and outcome. As a result, many theories have been constructed appropriate to various specific foci of observations or levels of interest. These necessitate different techniques of study, for which expertise in various scientific disciplines is required. Each requires concentration, technology and language specific for its purposes. Yet each is dependent on others especially on clinical or empirical investigations to define what is being studied. The geneticist, biochemist or physiologist, etc. requires firm and accurate diagnoses to be sure he is studying processes of schizophrenics, their subcategories and the state or phase of the everchanging disturbance.

For example, the combined experiences and study of the literature by several psychologists and psychiatrists years ago forced us into an artificial consensus to develop a Michael Reese definition of schizophrenia as a temporary working hypothesis, as stated before. What is needed now is a well-conceived program of study *in continuity* to define clinical schizophrenia and its categories, that can be useful for all scientific studies. Briefly stated, I believe that this requires a study of verbal and gross behaviors in relatively free fields where opportunities are present for many kinds of relations with a variety of people. The focus then would be on what challenges, well-defined, excite or ameliorate equally well-defined categories of responses? What psychological tests represent these challenges in brief or miniature encounters?

When we know more about what schizophrenia and/or its categories are, then geneticists, physiologists, chemists, psychologists and sociologists will be studying the same process. Certainly all subsystems, but some more than others (genetics), require behavioral referents for their correlations. Yet today we know that simple correlations artificially disregard different units of measurement and different temporal dimensions. Modern multivariate analyses require clinical phenomena and classifications as the scientific backbone on which the flesh of a host of other variables may be properly positioned.

We have become increasingly aware that correlations between brain-structure function and behavior, between emotional affective responses and internal feelings and concerns, between deficient logical structures and capacities for abstract thinking, between limited emotional and cognitive means and adaptation to reality are indeed not simple.[9] As a result, more interest in *bridging theories and models* has developed.

It is not that we should discard theories appropriate to various levels of organization and experience, nor abolish specific methods of investigation. Indeed, it is perfectly reasonable to assume that, though the many parts of the psychiatric *research system* may function harmoniously under control, at times one or the other discipline may dominate depending on the breakthrough of new information in that field. Over time there will be a considerable variation in the amount and relevance of productivity in one of the part-disciplines. In general, the permutations may be expressed by the syllogism: "If so and so and so, but not so and so then—."

To put each area of study in an appropriate position within a total field, so that the transactions among its parts may be defined in process-terms by observations from several specific frames of reference, then permits a larger more *integrative* view of the total biopsychosocial system.

REFERENCES

1. Bertalanffy, L. General systems theory and psychiatry. In S. Arieti (Ed.) *American handbook of psychiatry.* Vol. III. New York: Basic Books, 1966.
2, Gray, W., Duhl, F. J., & Rizzo, N. D. (Eds.) *General systems theory and psychiatry.* Boston: Little, Brown, 1969.
3. Ruesch, J. General systems theory based on human communications. In W. Gray, F. J. Duhl, N. D. Rizzo, (Eds.), *op. cit.,* 1969.
4. Grinker, R. R., Sr. Comparison of psychological "repression" and neurological "inhibition." *Journ. Nerv. & Ment. Dis.,* 1954, **89**, 765.
5. Grinker, R. R., Sr. An essay on schizophrenia and science. *Arch. Gen. Psych.,* 1969, **20**, 1–24.
6. Meehl, P. Schizotaxis, schizotypy and schizophrenia. *American Psychologist,* 1956, **17**, 827.
7. Grinker, R. R., Sr. Anxiety as a significant variable for a unified theory of human behavior. *Arch. Gen. Psych.,* 1959, **1**, 537–546.

8. Bleuler, E. The physiogenetic and psychogenic in schizophrenia. *Amer. Journ. Psychiatry*, 1930, **87**, 203–211.
9. Bleuler, M. A 23-year longitudinal study of 208 schizophrenics and impressions in regard to the nature of schizophrenia. In D. Rosenthal & S. S. Kety (Eds.), *The transmission of schizophrenia.* Oxford, England: Pergamon Press, 1968.
10. Lewis, A. Manfred Bleuler: The schizophrenic mental disorder—an exposition and a review. *Psychological Medicine*, 1973, **3**, 385–392.
11. Grinker, R. R., Sr., & Holzman, P. S. Schizophrenic pathology in young adults. *Arch. Gen. Psych.*, 1973, **28**, 168–175.
12. Apter, N. Our growing restlessness with problems of chronic schizophrenia. In L. Appleby, J. M. Scher, & J. Cummings (Eds.), *Chronic schizophrenia.* New York: The Free Press of Glencoe, 1960.
13. Beck, S. J. *The six schizophrenias.* New York: Grune & Stratton, 1953.
14. Macfie Campbell, C. *Destiny and disease in mental disorders with special reference to the schizophrenic psychoses.* New York: W. W. Norton, 1935.
15. Jones, F. H. Current methodologies for studying the development of schizophrenia. A critical review. *Journ. Nerv. and Mental Diseases*, 1973, **157**, 154–175.
16. Harrow, M., Harkay, K., Bromet, E., & Tucker, G. J. A longitudinal study of schizophrenic thinking. *Arch. Gen. Psych.*, 1973, **28**, 179–182.
17. Harrow, M., Tucker, G., Himmelboch, J., & Putnam, N. Schizophrenic thought disorders after the acute phase. *Amer. Journ. Psych.*, 1972, **128**, 58–63.
18. Astrachan, B. M., Harrow, M., Adler, L., Brawer, A., Schwartz, A., Schwartz, C., & Tucker, G. A checklist for the diagnosis of schizophrenia. *British Journ. of Psychiatry*, 1972, **121**, 529–539.
19. Holzman, P. A. *Neurobiological aspects of psychopathology.* New York: Grune & Stratton, 1969.
20. Epstein, S., & Coleman, M. Drive theories and schizophrenia. *Psychosomatic Medicine*, 1970, **32**, 113–140.
21. Sankar, D. V. S. (Ed.) *Schizophrenia: current concepts and research.* Hicksville: P. J. D. Publications, 1969.

22. Kallmann, F. J. *Heredity in health and mental disorder.* New York: W. W. Norton, 1953.
23. Rosenthal, D. Problems of sampling and diagnosis in the major twin studies of schizophrenia. *Journ. of Psychiatric Research,* 1961, **1**, 116–134.
24. Rosenthal, D., & Kety, S. S. *Transmission of schizophrenia.* New York: Pergamon Press, 1968.
25. Kringlen, Einar. Heredity and environment in the functional psychoses. Vol. I. *An epidemiological-clinical twin study.* Vol. II, Case histories. Oslo: Universitetsforlaget, 1968. Also *Psychiatry,* 1966, **29**, 172–184.
26. Kety, S. S., Rosenthal, D., Wender. P. H., & Schulsinger, W. The types and prevalence of mental illness in the biological and adoptive families of adopted schizophrenics. *Journ. Psychiatric Research,* 1968, **6**, 345–362.
27. Schildkraut, J. J., & Kety, S. Biogenic amines and emotions. *Science,* 1956, **156**, 21–30.
28. Ciba Foundation Symposium 8 (new series). *Physiology, emotions and psychosomatic illness.* North Holland, Elsevier: Excerpta Medica, 1972.
29. Ban, T. A. *Recent advances in the biology of schizophrenia.* Springfield, Ill.: Charles C Thomas, 1973.
30. Heath, R. Brain centers and control of behavior in man. In J. Nodine & J. H. Mayer (Eds.) *Psychosomatic medicine.* Philadelphia: Lea and Febiger.
31. Frohman, C. E., Harmison, C. R., Arthur, R. E., & Gottleib, J. C. Confirmation of a unique plasma protein in schizophrenia. *Biol. Psychiatry,* 1971, **3**, 113–121.
32. Calloway, E., Jones, R. T., & Layne, R. S. Evoked responses and segmental set of schizophrenia. *Arch. Gen. Psych.,* 1965, **12**, 83–89.
33. Giannitrapani, D., & Kayton, L. Schizophrenia and EEG spectral analysis. *Electroencephalography and Clinical Neurophysiology,* 1974, **36**, 377–386.
34. Grinker, R. R., Sr. A method for studying and influencing corticohypothalamic relations. *Science,* 1938, **87**, 73–74.
35. Grinker, R. R., Sr., & Serota, H. M. Electroencephalographic studies of corticohypothalamic relations in schizophrenia. *Amer. Jour. of Psych.,* 1941, **98**, 385–392.

36. Holzman, P. S., Procter, H., & Hughes, J. Eye tracking patterns in schizophrenia. *Science,* 1973, **181,** 179–181.
37. Spohn, H. E., Thetford, P. E., & Cancro, R. Attention, psychophysiology, and scanning in schizophrenic syndrome. In R. Cancro (Ed.), *The schizophrenic reactions.* New York: Brunner/Mazel, 1970.
38. Burnham, D. L. Varieties of reality restructuring in schizophrenia. In R. Cancro (Ed.), *The schizophrenic reactions.* New York: Brunner/Mazel, 1970.
39. Shakow, D. Some general comments and introductory remarks to the panel discussion. In R. Cancro (Ed.), *The schizophrenic reactions.* New York: Brunner/Mazel, 1970.
40. Grinker, R. R., Sr. Diagnosis and schizophrenia. In R. Cancro (Ed.), *The schizophrenic reactions.* New York: Brunner/Mazel, 1970.
41. Mishler, E. G., & Waxler, N. E. Family interaction processes and schizophrenia: a review of current theories. *Int. Journ. of Psychiatry,* 1966, **2,** 375.
42. Lidz, T. *The origin and treatment of schizophrenic disorders.* New York: Basic Books, 1973.
43. Wynne, L. C. Family transactions and schizophrenia. In J. Romano (Ed.), *The origins of schizophrenia.* Amsterdam: Excerpta Medica, 1967.
44. Anthony, E. J. A clinical evaluation of children with psychotic parents. *Amer. Journ. Psych.,* 1969, **26,** 117–184.
45. Grinker, R. R., Sr. The effect of infantile disease on ego patterns. *Amer. Journ. Psych.,* 1941. **98,** 385–392.
46. Bender, L. Twenty years of clinical research on schizophrenia with special reference to those under 6 years of age. *Journal of Autism and Childhood Schizophrenia,* 1971, **1,** 115–118.
47. Escalona, S., & Heider, G. M. *Prediction and outcome.* New York: Basic Books, 1959.
48. Brody, S. *Patterns of mothering.* New York: International Universities Press, 1956.
49. Gesell, A., & Amatruda, C. *The embryology of behavior.* New York: Harper, 1945.
50. Rieder, R. O. The offspring of schizophrenic parents: a review. *Journ. Nerv. and Mental Dis.,* 1973, **157,** 179.

51. Shakow, D. Schizophrenic research and high risk studies. *Psychiatry*, 1973, **36**, 353–366.
52. Robins, L. N. *Deviant children grown up.* Baltimore: Williams and Wilkins, 1966.
53. Shakow, D. Some observations on the psychology (and some fewer on the biology) of schizophrenia. *Journ. Nerv. Ment. Dis.*, 1971, **153**, 300–316.
54. Koh, S., Kayton, L., & Berry, R. Mnemonic organization in young nonpsychotic schizophrenics. *Journ. Abnormal Psychol.*, 1973, **81**, 289–310.
55. Koh, S. D., & Kayton, L. Memorization of word strings by young nonpsychotic psychophrenics. *Journ. of Abnormal Psychology*, 1974, **83**, 14–23.
56. Dunham, H. W. Sociocultural studies of schizophrenia. *Arch. Gen. Psych.*, 1971, **24**, 206–214.
57. Yi-Chiang, L. Contradictory parental expectations in schizophrenia. Dependence and responsibility. *Arch. Gen. Psych.*, 1962, **6**, 219–234.
58. Bellak, L., & Loeb, L. *The schizophrenic syndrome.* New York: Grune & Stratton, 1969.
59. Romano, J. (Ed.) *The origins of schizophrenia.* Amsterdam: Excerpta Medica, 1967.
60. Jackson, D. D. (Ed.) *The etiology of schizophrenia.* New York: Basic Books, 1960.
61. Holley, J. W., & Nilsson, J. K. On the validity of some clinical measures. *Psychological Research Bulletin* (Published by Lund Universities Press, Lund, Sweden), 1973, **13**, 4.

XIV

The Role of Psychiatry in Society

All sciences, including their primitive precursor, mythology,[1] are closely involved in their contemporary social matrix, either directly or indirectly. Psychiatry is, in part, a social science, since man is a social animal during health or illness, and his individuality is only approximate, not ultimate. Society demands, requests, condones and condemns some forms of psychiatry, just as it deals with other intellectual trends in its component members or groups. In this sense, psychiatry is *in* society. In another sense, psychiatry and society are two systems closely related to each other by way of transactions between their interfaces. The interface between society and medicine, including psychiatry, is stated clearly by Charles Johnson:[2] "Social sciences furnish foundations which enable psychiatry to link medicine with social situations within the broad control of culture." To understand this relationship one has to designate those parts of society with which psychiatry exchanges informa-

This chapter is an abbreviated and modified version of a paper presented at the 200th anniversary of the Williamsburg State Psychiatric Hospital in West Virginia, October 10, 1973, with permission of Dr. George Kriegman.

tion. These include the family, the neighborhood and other geographical partitions, the school, police, church, work, etc.

Until humans accept the "mankind" concept with its over arching, all-embracing recognition of a conspecies, society as a global concept has little practical or operational value. On the other hand, one of psychiatry's major problems is its vagueness, diffusion and confusion of terms. The field's vocabulary is neither consensual within its own boundaries, nor with bordering systems, and we correctly are accused of speaking and writing in jargon. Even within the field, terms are not adequately defined in theory or operations. Think of the many words borrowed from physics such as "psychic energy," or quantitative statements such as "cathexis" or "neutralization of aggressive energy."

Joseph Fletcher[3] defines positive human criteria as: minimal intelligence, self-consciousness, self-control, a sense of time, a sense of the future and the past, concern for others, communications with others, control of existence, curiosity, change and changeability, balance of rationality and feeling. He states that good answers to the question of the nature of man, "are more apt to be found inductively and empirically from medical science and the clinicians than by the necessarily syllogistic reasoning of the humanities."

Obviously, within Fletcher's simple, easily understandable statements there are no connotations of "positive mental health."[4] However, in considering psychiatry and society, we cannot avoid discussing the heavily value-laden and biased concepts of health, normality and illness. Strupp[5] defines health and illness as follows: "The normal has come to terms with problems of social illness and has succeeded in modulating it, the neurotic continues to make an issue of it and the psychopath turns his back on it." Whitehorn and Betz[6] state that the healthy person loves well, plays well, works well and expects well (cf. Chapter VII).

Society determines what is mental health for its population.[7] When, in Mell's cartoon, Ira's teacher asked him, "Ira, don't you want to be known as a normal, average, American boy?" He answered, "No, I want to be like all the others." Health is a value system dependent on the place, time and population. Each set of conditions imposes a threshold beyond which deviance becomes intolerable and is termed illness. Anselm Strauss *et al.*[8] have stated: "We need much more sophistication about normality—a sociological range and differentiation of normal behavior now almost altogether missing in the psychiatrist's thinking."

Society not only lays down standards of health and the acceptance of the secondary role of illness, but also the means by which coping mechanisms may be used in the stresses of development, which seem to be phase specific, and in the threatening events and crises in our turbulent lives.

> Normality and illness are only polarities of a wide range of integrations—when strained the organismic systems respond according to the processes by which the many subvariances have become integrated—thus, the degree of health and illness in the stress-responses reveals the quality and quantity of integration.[9]

Having indicated so far the close relationship between psychiatry and society, we now attempt to define, not psychiatry, but the *multiple* psychiatries as they have evolved and exist today. The lay public has come to think of psychiatrists as doctors practicing a branch of medicine. This indeed they do, although after medical school and graduate education most of them promptly forget all they have learned about the body, refusing to touch it as if it were abhorrent. For the higher socioeconomic classes, a psychiatrist is someone who uses words or interpretations almost exclusively, and is called a *psychotherapist.*

Psychotherapy is old. Hippocrates relied on expectations that the baths, rest, beautiful climate and general environment at his hospital would cure many. The witch doctors of Africa still, after years of training, use impressive surroundings, strange intruments, unintelligible words and high fees to achieve good results. Indeed, the nonspecific elements of all therapies seem to be the crucial factors for recovery. Each school of therapy uses its own methods for everything. Who directs the patient to which and why?

It is indeed true that psychotherapy, dynamic or otherwise, is a dominant treatment modality in psychiatry that is conducted by physicians who practice this specialty, but this has been reinforced by a segment of society's acceptance and demands. More than that, psychiatrists have influenced social work therapists, clinical psychologists and, latterly, nurses to conduct individual, group and family psychotherapy.

Another group of psychiatrists are called *somatotherapists* because they adhere strictly to the medical model, thus utilizing electric shock whenever possible and a wide range of drugs. These drugs include the antischizophrenic and antidepressive compounds, as well as lithium for manic attacks, singly or in combination. True, they say they also do psychotherapy, but greeting and a few kind words can hardly deserve such a term. On the other hand, psychotherapists are becoming increasingly willing to use drugs as adjuncts and facilitators for their own brand of therapy This was not always so, because when the phenothiazines first appeared, Sabshin and Ramot[10] reported that the psychotherapists at our hospital were reluctant to use drugs or used them in insufficient doses. The entire social field composed of doctors and nurses was biased against the use of drugs, and during the 1950's, the results were less positive than elsewhere. Now, with a strongly positive bias, the social field reinforces the value of medication to the extent that it has become more difficult to evaluate the effect of any form of treatment by itself.

Another interaction between society and psychiatric therapists is the treatment of patients of lower socioeconomic status when the patients are in crises. Many psychiatrists have the idea that such patients are not suitable for psychotherapy, which is not true. But many of these patients, considering that the psychiatrists are doctors, demand medication at once and are in a hurry to leave the hospital to return to job and/or home. Once away, it is extremely difficult to persuade them to continue treatment on an outpatient basis.

A third group of psychiatrists may be called *sociotherapists*, in that they emphasize milieu therapy in the hospital and group or family therapy both for inpatients and outpatients. They, more than the others, veer away from the medical model, although not to the extent that Albee[11] recommends; not only is their treatment modality nonmedical, but they denigrate diagnostic terms and specific therapies. Instead, they repudiate the concept of illness, substituting for it "disturbances resulting from problems in living." Society has in part accepted this distinction and has become enamored with so called "encounter" groups, to the dismay of many of us.

An altogether different social form of therapy is conducted by the existentialist, who bases his approach on the philosophy of Kierkegaard.[12] The existential psychiatrist attempts to help his patients who are afraid of not being free to find themselves, except by dichotomizing themselves and the social, economic world to which they are bound on this earth. But they cannot leave through hallucinatory drugs or by living in isolated communes. They can only be free selves as part of the society in which they live.

The three models[8] that have been described correspond to the definition of psychiatry as a medical specialty devoted to the diagnosis and treatment of mental illness. The sharpness of the separation among them is increasingly becoming blurred. But diagnostic criteria and, for that matter, interest in diagnosis are deficient, so that therapy in psychiatry cannot be considered even as an applied science. Yet, in a psychology conference on graduate education held in the 1940's, it was said that psychotherapy is an undefined technic applied to unspecified problems with unpredictable results. For this technic rigorous training was recommended!

What, then, is the science of psychiatry, if there is such a field? How is it different from the delivery of services for which there is little enquiry or evaluation? Society is interested in services, and often in instant results, but how do we learn more about human problems in order to satisfy the needs and demands of society? It is relevant at this point to quote from Daniel X. Freedman's[13] cogent essay:

> Such a society, especially a technological society, would come to value science as a social system through which the understanding of nature and human nature is advanced. They would, on reflection, appreciate that this happens through a mode of activities that conserves, adjudicates, accumulates and transforms knowledge, a mode that transcends the ability of single individuals as well as generations. The business of doing this involves investigators, doers and appliers. It involves scholars who look back for perspective and critical teachers who, comprehending the contingent status of knowledge, equip the young for the unknown future. Such a system incidentally goes against our intrinsic megalomanic and wishful trends. It requires some valuing of objectivity and the ability to see the unwanted, to be jolted from custom and belief, to tolerate ambiguity and delay of gratification in pursuit of the future, and to enjoy such disci-

pline and insecurity for the intellectual payoff and, once in a while, for the actual practical gain. Such values conserve knowledge but they also underwrite, expect and anticipate change. Such values challenge our imperfections while perfecting our mastery of them.

James Frazer,[1] in his masterful *The Golden Bough,* described the common primitive roots of science and magic, both of which follow general rules. Magic developed into religion with belief in powers higher than man. These powers must be propitiated in true faith—just as much now as millennia ago—whether they be gods or God, drugs, leaders of the various social systems that are now springing up as multiple aberrant communes or singularly led encounter groups, or even existential faith in self. Much magic persists in psychiatry, but society's faith in its powers has waned, and in many places the faith has turned to overt and covert contempt.

Mysticism has taken two general forms. One is the emphasis on a new humanism; even a mutation[14] of consciousness to an integration of a "perspective world." The other is a mystical overevaluation of a human figure, making him into a faultless God—as Eissler[15] does to Freud.

Sometime in the latter part of the 1950's, research and clinical psychiatrists became self-conscious when they suddenly discovered that psychiatry was an integral part of the vast field of the behavioral sciences.[16] Their focus could no longer block out larger areas of behavior such as the biological, psychological, social or economic. Ideas of unified or systems theory seemed to furnish answers in their concepts of openness, communications, transations, homeostasis and isomorphism. Thus, on the one hand, clinical psychiatry began to participate in social action under increased political freedom and, on the other hand, research psychiatry absorbed field theories.

When we think of society, and of psychiatry as a science in the modern sense of systems, it is possible to think of psychiatry as part of the social system which is composed of many other parts. Thus, the larger social system may condone, condemn or support change, recognizing research as fulfilling the need to search and to change our notion of man and enhance the quality of living.

A more productive way of looking at psychiatry as a system,[17] in order to preclude setting up dichotomies between reductionism and/or humanness, is to represent the sciences of sociology and anthropology as parts of the psychiatric system.

We conceive of psychiatry as a biopsychosocial system which[18] attempts to synthesize behavioral sciences into a unified theory of human behavior. It is an important fact that social and personality components are interdependent and interpenetrate. All parts constitute an organization which is controlled and regulated by the unifying principle of survival or homeostasis which encompasses stability, growth, evolution, social organization, increasing complexity and optimum variability.[19]

We are becoming increasingly aware of the reciprocal relationship between personality characteristics that, under proper conditions, predispose an individual to the full-blown disorder, disease or deviance (whichever name is a matter of choice). This reciprocal movement is clear in the depressive,[20] borderline[21] and schizophrenics.[22] From disease state back to character traits is the most that can be hoped for from any therapy.

Our concepts of the multiple causes of emotional and cognitive disturbances and their treatment are certainly dependent on our view as observers of the transactions between social, personality and cultural processes. Are personality deviances due to difficult or traumatic experiences in early family life? How much do conflicts in society contribute to psychological malfunctioning? We have begun to realize that phases of the lifecycle encounter different social problems: several phases of childhood, adolescence, young adulthood, adulthood and aging.

Likewise, society is not a uniform process. Ours is not a unitary society as the "melting pot" mythology indicates. Indeed, it is a pluralistic society composed of various ethnic groups, socioeconomic classes and colors. Our states and regions are still differentiated by their geography, resources and industries. Our so-called two-party political system indeed reveals its coalition composition, in that the parties are held together by the character of their leaders.

Just as we cannot speak of *a* psychiatry, we cannot speak of *a* society. Where a person is born, where he lives, is educated and works exposes him to different societies and cultures which make demands on him and to which he must adapt. Moving from one place to another, even so short a distance as from a city to its suburbs, or destroying a neighborhood to build a throughway, requires a different form of coping.

Thus we have systems in process in constant movement with individuals growing, maturing, developing into different phases of the lifecycle; society changing with incredible speed due to technological discoveries. A one-to-one relationship, a matching between personality or psychopathy and socio-cultural factors is thus very difficult. This has always been so, although psychiatrists have ignored the rapidly shifting internal and external factors involved in psychiatry. Recognition now results in less certainty, albeit greater sophistication in research, as controlling for many variables has become more difficult.

So far we have discussed psychiatry and society as systems with their own parts and regulatory functions, interpenetrating so that one can become part of the other and vice versa, or so that they may transact as separate systems. But society has little regard for the conceptual and abstract, or investment in its future. Immediate action is demanded.

Drugs appropriate for specific conditions are ingested universally in order to "feel better." Behavioral therapy short-cuts insight and freedom is sacrificed in order to be shaped into desirable molds. American social fickleness is portrayed by its rapid shift of bandwagons.[23]

We are still being influenced by the big-business government's attitude as stated by Charles Wilson of General Motors, who said that basic research is when you don't know what you are doing. So we are asked to do target research or research of relevance. But who knows what is relevant and where the target is? Nobelist Szent-Gyorgyi tells the story of how his faked projects were supported and his realistic projects were rejected by the "Popes of the field." Psychiatrists are not social engineers. Neither are they politicians able to lobby well for their own purposes nor do they do well with the local community's Board of Directors. Statements of opinion about social issues should be made only by psychiatrists as citizens. Official and professional opinions are only for the purpose of advising on procedures to further mental health and point out what actions are detrimental.

We have become misled by our own professional bureaucrats who have assumed a political role as advisors to the various governmental agencies. They assume that they speak for the workers in the field. Promises of prevention have been made for as long as we can remember. Curing everybody by anything seems to be accepted by the public each time a new name is invented. The profession has been split by bureaucrats belaboring a "private sector," when indeed most practitioners hold part-time jobs and most psychiatrists working in public hospitals do part-time practice.

We do have grave responsibilities, as does all of medicine, toward society, transcending our specific professionalism, which is dedicated to preserving and improving human life. Once we tamper with the right to live for all, no matter what the cost, we sacrifice our democratic way of life and would eventually degenerate into a genocidal culture. Yet there are ethical problems raised by the Hastings Institute. These include death and dying, behavioral control, population policy and genetic counseling.

There is a more pressing ethical issue for psychiatrists over and above keeping the mentally retarded and the hopelessly senile alive. With increasing confidence that there is a biological basis to the development of the schizophrenic system, we should be aware that we are increasing the genetic pool by the use of antischizophrenic drugs, discharge from warehouses, enabling marriage and child bearing.

A recent Ciba Foundation Conference,[24] although not containing any reference to psychiatry nor having a single psychiatric participant, discussed the current anti-scientific movement, blaming scientists for ruining the golden age of mankind. Today science is tolerated only if socially relevant, and scientists are criticized for lack of social responsibilities and lack of values. There is a movement to evaluate and control science in terms of its relevance. Science is considered to be in conflict with humanism, ignoring individuality, imagination, quality and the concrete. A plea is being made for a framework of institutional policy-making in the interest of the nonscientific majority.

The American humanistic psychologists and existential psychiatrists are mostly closer to the psychodynamicists than they are to Sartre:

> Their clinical experiences have led them to conceive of the human being as having an essence, a biological nature, membership in a species. It is very easy to interpret the "uncovering" therapies as helping the person to discover his Identity, his "Real Self," in a word, his own subjective biology, which he can then proceed to actualize, to "make himself," to "choose." The Freudian conception of instincts has been gener-

ally discarded by the humanistic psychologists in favor of the conception of "basic needs," or in some cases, in favor of the conception of a single overarching need for actualization or growth. In any case, it is implied, if not made explicit, by most of these writers that the organism, in the strictest sense, has needs which must be gratified in order to become fully human, to grow well, and to avoid sicknesses. This doctine of a "Real Self" to be uncovered and actualized is also a total rejection of the tabula rasa notions of the behaviorists and associationists who often talk as if anything can be learned, anything can be taught, as if the human being is a sort of a passive clay to be shaped, controlled, reinforced, modified in any way that somebody arbitrarily decides.

We speak then of a self, a kind of intrinsic nature which is very subtle, which is not necessarily conscious, which has to be sought for, and which has to be uncovered and then built upon, actualized, taught, educated. The notion is that something is there but it's hidden, swamped, distorted, twisted, overlayed. The job of the psychotherapist (or the teacher) is to help a person find out what's already in him rather than to reinforce him or shape or teach him into a prearranged form, which someone else has decided upon in advance, a priori [Maslow].[25]

According to Maslow,[25] there are two kinds of learning: extrinsic learning, given by teachers as possessions that we cherish, and personal learning, gained by experiences in becoming a human animal *similar* to others—a discovery *by ourselves* of our inner selves as *different* from others. It is learning to be a person, not the impersonal learning of skills. Maslow goes on to say:

The creative scientist then looks more like a gambler than a banker, one who is willing to work hard for seven years because of a dazzling hunch, one who feels certain in the absence of evidence, before the evidence, and only then proceeds to the hard work of proving or disproving his precious revelations. First comes the emotion, the fascination, the falling in love with a possibility, and then comes the hard work, the chores, the stubborn persistence in the face of disappointment and failure.

What is this conflict between science and humanism that has portrayed them as if they are two cultures? Maslow describes two types of science. One type may be called a kind of academic psychology derived from classical psychology theory. The second school, which could be called the philosophy of psychology, stems from the work of Freud; called psychodynamic or depth psychology, it generates theories of art, religion, society and almost every aspect of human endeavor.

Maslow contends that there is a third force in psychology:

> Third Force psychology, as some are calling it, is in large part a reaction to the gross inadequacies of behavioristic and Freudian psychologies in their treatment of the higher nature of man. Classical academic psychology has no systematic place for higher order elements of the personality such as altruism and dignity, or the search for truth and beauty. You simply do not ask questions about ultimate human values if you are working in an animal lab.

He discusses the higher needs of man: "needs" for the intrinsic and ultimate values of goodness and truth and beauty and perfection and justice and order. They exist and cannot be explained away that they represent illusions or defenses. Science, says Maslow, is not merely instrumental but is able to help mankind to discover its ultimate ends and values.

Herrick,[26] who was one of our great naturalists, states that science does not comprise all of human experience. Science, philosophy, esthetics, religion and all other domains of experience should cooperate harmoniously for a common objective—the enrichment of life. Faith includes the extension into the unknown. It is justifiable if it contributes to personal mental health and social betterment. Religion is the natural reaction of imagination when confronted with difficulties. "We may render to God the things that are God's and to science only the things that are nature's."

In sum, society in general and scientists in particular seem to be approaching the view that objectivity and subjectivity are inseparable and not in conflict. We all have a faith, more or less, in ourselves and in the future and yet, as well as we can, we follow the canons of objective science. The public as well should be taught of this necessary combination.

REFERENCES

1. Frazer, J. G. *The golden bough: a study in magic and religion.* Vol. 1. (3rd ed.) New York: Macmillan, 1935.
2. Johnson, C. S. The influence of social science on psychiatry. In R. R. Grinker, Sr. (Ed.), *Midcentury psychiatry.* Springfield, Ill.: Charles C Thomas, 1953, p. 144.
3. Fletcher, J. *Hastings center report.* Vol. 2. November, 1972.
4. Yahoda, M. *Current concepts of positive mental health.* New York: Basic Books, 1958.
5. Strupp, H. H. On the technic of psychotherapy. *Archives of General Psychiatry,* 1972, **26,** 270–278.
6. Whitehorn, J. C., & Betz, B. J. A comparison of psychotherapeutic relationship between physicians and schizophrenic patients. *American Journal of Psychiatry,* 1957, **113,** 901–910.
7. Grinker, R. R., Sr. Mentally healthy young males (homoclites). *Archives of General Psychiatry,* 1962, **6,** 404–453.

8. Strauss, A., Schatzman, L., Bucher, R., Ehrlich, D., & Sabshin, M. *Psychiatric ideologies and institutions.* New York: Free Press of Glencoe, 1964.
9. Grinker, R. R., Sr. Normality viewed as a system. *Archives of General Psychiatry,* 1967, **17,** 320–324.
10. Sabshin, M., & Ramot, J. Psychotherapeutic evaluation and the psychiatric setting. *Archives of Neurology and Psychiatry,* 1956, **75,** 362.
11. Albee, G. Emerging concepts of mental illness and models of treatment; the psychologist's point of view. *American Journal of Psychiatry,* 1969, **125,** 869. Also *Professional Psychology,* 1971, **2,** 128–145.
12. Beck, S. J. Either, Or. *Yale Review of Biology and Medicine,* 1972, **62,** 54–75.
13. Freedman, D. X. *Can we put research to work?* Highlights of the 17th annual conference of V. A. cooperative studies in mental health and the behavioral sciences, St Louis, March 1972.
14. Gerber, J. The foundations of the perspective world. Translated by K. F. Lerdecker. *Main Currents in Modern Thought,* 1972, **29,** 80–88.
15. Eissler, K. R. *Medical orthodoxy and the future of psychoanalysis.* New York: International Universities Press, 1965.
16. Luszki, M. D. (Ed.) *Interdisciplinary team research.* New York: New York University Press, 1958.
17. Grinker, R. R., Sr. "Open-system" psychiatry *American Journal of Psychoanalysis.* 1966, **26,** 115–128.
18. Grinker, R. R., Sr. The relevance of general systems theory of psychiatry. In D. A. Hamburg & H. K. H. Brodie (Eds., Vol. 6), *American handbook of psychiatry* (Overall ed. S. Arieti). New York: Basic Books, 1974.
19. Emerson, A. E. Dynamic homeostasis: a unifying principle in organic, social and ethical evolution. *Scientific Monthly,* 1954, **78,** 67–85.
20. Grinker, R. R., Sr., Miller, J., Sabshin, M., Nunn, R., & Nunnally, J. C. *The phenomena of depression.* New York: Hoeber, 1961.
21. Grinker, R. R., Sr., Werble, B., & Drye, R. C. *The borderline syndrome.* New York: Basic Books, 1968.

search but so-called basic research, conducted by scientists from those disciplines that form parts of the total psychiatric field or system. The history of scientific advances in all fields of medicine that ultimately spin off into concrete and valuable application to the human condition indicates the need for all forms of research, no matter how detached they seem at first from practical questions.

Unfortunately, the public has little patience, and its demands for crash programs that deliver immediate gains have been expressed by bureaucrats who advocate support of only "mission-oriented" research. The fact is, however, that achieving specific goals such as "community mental health"—a movement that promised primary prevention of mental illness—is still very far off in the future—if, indeed, it ever comes to pass, given the ever-present conflict between man's drives as an evolved animal and his socialized and cultural controls.

Similarly, psychiatrists have been seduced by, and even forced to accept, every new enterprise focused on treatment—to the neglect of theory, sound methods and systems of evaluation. As a result, psychiatry has been "riding madly in all directions."[2] The emphasis on quantity and equality of treatment for all has prematurely sacrificed the individuality of persons in trouble and seriously weakened sound scientific investigations. The misuse of new antischizophrenic, antidepressive and antimanic drugs has permeated widely for relief of almost any psychological complaint, just as the "miracle" antibiotics are demanded for conditions for which they are ineffective. These psychotropic drugs have and will continue to advance our knowledge of the biochemical constituents of cerebral activities as a part of the functional analysis of disorders involved in psychiatric diseases.

Furthermore, we have already witnessed the shifting nature of psychiatric entities in the last decades in that the dramatic, histrionic nature of neuroses and psychoses has decreased, except for delinquency and drug addiction.[3] Instead, humans attempting to cope with the strains of growth and development, and the response to failure and aging, are expressed more in terms of constriction and inhibition of personality and character. I believe that some aspects of our social and cultural surroundings are responsible, but I believe we need an investigation that will enlighten our current ignorance as to what elements are really responsible. The outward shifts in aberrant behavior in no way indicate that the quality of the human problems has changed.

The future of psychiatry hinges on changes that we cannot predict at this time in man's shifting behaviors in a changing society. For example, the wholesale increase in returning patients from state hospitals to the community may increase the biogenetic pool for psychosis and mental deficiency.

Shifts in family constellations from the extended to the nuclear family, increased urbanization, changes in the kind of parenting and other social and economic factors may result in changes in the kinds of coping available to succeeding generations.

Although epidemiology (which estimates the incidence and prevalence of mental illness, including illnesses that are not treated by therapy), and an estimation of the distribution of illness throughout various social classes are important methods for psychiatric research, we are confronted with problems of taxonomy or standardization of diagnosis. Many psychiatrists resist statistics and are fearful of psychiatric registries. Yet institutions must attempt what is as yet impossible—i.e., to document their utility.

We cannot reorganize society; we are novices in politics and we have not yet caught up sufficiently with the explosive progress in biological psychiatry to develop a modern neuropsychiatry. As Arthur[4] states:

Social psychiatry, which includes the study of the impingement of social phenomena upon the genesis, manifestations, and treatment of mental and physical illness, has in recent decades become an increasingly important part of psychiatry. The epidemiology and taxonomy of mental illness, social factors in the onset and course of disease, transcultural psychiatry are all fields that have shown great expansion. But the results of the experiences of community psychiatry and of social psychiatric studies have played a major role in the development of a crisis of identity within the profession of psychiatry; the appropriate education and professional activities for a psychiatrist are currently in dispute.

All of this means that psychiatry is necessarily part of the process of change, at least in diagnosis, treatment and possibly in preventive measures. All the more reason why solid, well-designed research in all disciplines of psychiatry should be supported and greatly extended if our civilization does not nurture the seeds of its own destruction. We can no longer afford the luxury of making public generalizations for the narcissistic purpose of appearing to be an expert. Those who treat should treat adequately for the problems of our difficult lives, and those who investigate should be free to explore with adequate support that which needs to be researched.

Brodie and Sabshin[5] reviewed the number and types of research articles published in the *Archives of General Psychiatry* and the *American Journal of Psychiatry* during the last decade. At the beginning of the decade the emphasis on research was weak (37 per cent of the papers), but by the end of 1972 it had increased to 48 per cent. However, declining governmental support may reverse this trend in the next decade. In the order of the biopsychosocial system, biological research (genetics) was most frequent, psychological research took second place, and sociological research was third. In the order of kinds of topics, mechanisms (dynamics) came first, therapy (biological) second and etiology third.

Astrup[6] states:

> There is, however, a need for physiological explanations of how social and psychological factors act on the mind. This may be formulated through conditioning and other psychophysiological studies. The importance of developing objective, comparatively "culture-free" methods for international comparisons of impairment of mental health should not be forgotten. The lack of such methods in the vast literature of social psychiatric field-studies from all parts of the world may be one factor contributing to the great difficulty one encounters in comparing the findings of various authors.
>
> It would be of particularly great interest to follow children from birth up to the age when adult neuroses and psychoses begin to appear. But this would imply more than a follow-up for a single generation. Results of short-term projects of five to ten years could best be obtained in limited populations with "normal" age distributions, so that even a prophylaxis of senile psychoses could be elaborated.
>
> In attacking the problem of prevention of mental illness, a large number of approaches must be used. This implies that several centers from many countries will have to combine their know-how in order to adequately utilize the present state of knowledge and theory.

The future of research in psychiatry cannot rest with the current generation of investigators because they are too few and are decreasing by attrition. The future rests on goals and methods of educational process to which the young aspirants are exposed. Unfortunately, there are many obstacles based on outside pressures over which we have limited control.

There is currently a mad rush in professional education that squeezes the time allotted for training to absurd proportions. The development of three-year medical schools and the abolition of the internship period forces the student to choose a specialization long before he has had sufficient life experiences to mature and develop. He then is confronted by psychiatry's rapid extension into areas of prevention that should more properly concern public health physicians and sociologists. In fact, Cerrolza[7] writes about the "psychiatrization of life," paraphrasing an earlier statement of mine that psychiatry has extended to include all of life.

The masters hovering over our academic functions, especially psychiatry—the groups that tell us what we should teach and research—are the governmental funding bodies, both national and local, that use the threat of withholding support. As Romano[8] points out, the bureaucrats, with their misguided concepts of medical ethics, have established rules and regulations regarding "informed consent" that have stifled much needed psychiatric research, research that can be carried out without the slightest harm to the patient. Because a few investigators have performed ill-advised and badly controlled research, the whole field has had to suffer, especially in the areas of stress and drug research.

Most training institutions can give a smattering or taste of parts of general psychiatry, while few can encompass the whole field. There is very little time adequately to teach a specialty within the field, and there are now many such specialties.

So far as research is concerned this book has touched on many problems—including the functions and make-up of the researcher. But the individual investigator is now virtually extinct. He needs a multidisciplinary team, as the following passages make explicit.

Blatt[9] states:

war, about the adaptability of social classes, or about
the malleability of individual beings, except for those
frail generalizations that we assemble from our real
and vicarious experience—itself biased by our situation within society and our private predilections.
Thus, to the most important element of an effort to
assess the prospect for man we have no guide but
ourselves, and are thrown back to criteria that trouble
us by virtue of their subjective foundation.

In the preface of this book I indicated a reluctance to
view the changing psychiatric scene through episodes of
my life. In spite of this decision, the questions of what
makes a researcher and where the future of psychiatry lies,
seem somehow related to personal experiences. At the urg-
ing of some of my friends, I therefore decided to offer a
brief summary of my own career as a prototype.

I was the first son, and the first grandchild, born of a
mother who devoted her life to her children and her home.
My father, forced to make out for himself from the age of
13, had a difficult youth. He became a neuropsychiatrist
almost by accident, but he worked hard, studied constantly,
and became a successful clinician. He was also a scholar,
and accumulated an extensive library containing a wide
variety of books on every subject, including neurology and
psychiatry. These books were my friends, with whom I
spent every afternoon sprawled on the floor of the library.
My father was an excellent teacher, and he wrote exten-
sively on specific case-reports, which were what constituted
research at that time.

Father and son talked about problems of the world at the
dinner table and during weekly walks in the park. I learned
logic and concise manners of describing and defining conclusions from our observations. Scholarly pursuits opened
up a fantastic world to discover and to understand. At the
same time, his friends burdened me with the expectation
that I was to be better than father, which created a heavy

load to bear for the future; and, indeed, troubles were in store for me.

Zoology in high school was impossible because I couldn't identify birds, not knowing that my difficulty stemmed from the fact that I was color-blind. My medical career was almost ruined when I flunked physics in premedical school because of my complete lack of mathmatical ability. My B.S. degree was delayed two years because of my aversion to exercise. In medical school, I couldn't figure out how the baby should be turned to facilitate its exit from the birth canal. But, finally I made it and graduated from Rush Medical School and passed the examination for internship at the Cook County Hospital.

My father supported me after my marriage for a year abroad of postgraduate studies in neurology. Two things were important: 1) I came in contact with great men in the field of neurology—Marburg, Monakow, Jakob, Gordon Holmes, Kinnier Wilson and Walsh; and 2) my wife, who has been my wife now for 50 years, agreed to let me work five nights a week and I in turn agreed to become involved socially during the other two, doing anything she wished. It worked!

Returning to the University of Chicago after my father died, I worked with Percival Bailey in the Division of Neurology and Neurosurgery. He was an inspiration for me. After several years I was asked to take a Rockefeller Fellowship to develop psychiatry at the University. In preparation for the work, I was analysed by Freud, visited all the German universities and worked at the Psychiatric Institute in London under Maypother, Aubrey Lewis, Crichley and Carmichael; I also stopped off at Hopkins to listen to Adolph Meyer. During the course of these explorations, I learned a good deal about psychiatry.

But things did not go well at the University and after a few years, at the request of Michael Reese, I left to set up a psychiatric unit there. Shortly afterwards, I spent three years in the Air Forces, overseas and in Florida, during which period I became adept at extemporaneous speaking and wrote two books with my ex-resident John P. Spiegel (one was *Men Under Stress*). When we returned to Michael Reese, a new Psychiatric Institute had been planned and in 1951 we opened it—despite my great apprehension about my ability to do the job as director. That I succeeded is still a surprise to me. I still work hard, have optimism for the future and plan on retiring only by force of illness. My current program of research aided by several excellent colleagues will certainly not be finished during my lifetime, but it is started and I at least enjoy its beginnings.

What does this all mean? What generalization can be made from this brief account of one man's life, since others may achieve much more on the basis of different circumstances? Let me enumerate them: A good genetic inheritance, a paternal model of scholarship, a compulsive dedication to excellence (with oneself, not the world, as one's most severe critic), a mother whose love I was certain about, a wife who partook of and belonged to my career, an opportunity for excellent training, an unslaked curiosity that led to research as a way of life, accidental encounters that furthered a research career (fellowships, University appointment, an Institute with adequate resources) good people to work for and with, and good people to train.

I know that there are many other ways by which many others may insure the future of psychiatry. I did what I had to do based on my past: the external pressures that eventually became internalized. It was hard work and there was lots of suffering, but the end is worth it and I hope that just as my students—John Spiegel, George Ham, Louis Robbins, Louis Gottschalk, David Hamburg, Melvin Sabshin, Donald Oken, Daniel Offer, Edward Wolpert, Larry Kayton, Michael Basch, Alvin Suslick, John Gedo, Arnold Goldberg and others—have contributed to the future of psychiatry, others will also do so.

I close this chapter and book with a passage that Bertrand Russell[13] wrote almost 25 years ago; a passage that is optimistic and that also expresses a somber note of warning:

> The near future must be either much better or much worse than the past; which it is to be I do not know, but those of you who are still young will know before very long (p. 14).

REFERENCES

1. Offer, D., & Freedman, D. X. *Modern psychiatry and clinical research.* New York: Basic Books, 1972.
2. Grinker, R. R., Sr. Psychiatry rides madly in all directions. *Arch. Gen. Psych.*, 1964, **10**, 228.
3. Grinker, R. R., Sr., Schimel, J. L., Salzman, L., Chodoff, P., & Will, O. Changing styles in psychiatric syndromes. *American Journal Psychiatry*, 1973, 130, 147–155.
4. Arthur, R. J. Social psychiatry: an overview. *Navy Medical Neuropsychiatric Research Unit, Report #73–74.* Washington, D.C., 1973.
5. Brodie, H. K. H., & Sabshin, M. An overview of trends in psychiatric research 1963–1972. *American Journal Psychiatry*, 1973, **130**, 1309–1318.
6. Astrup, C. Proposal for a prophylactic psychiatry. *Biological Psychiatric*, 1973, **6**, 107–108.
7. Cerrolza, M. The nebulous scope of current psychiatry. *Comprehensive Psychiatry* 1973, **14**, 299–309.
8. Romano, J. Reflections on informed consent. *Arch. Gen. Psych.*, 1974, **30**, 129–135.
9. Blatt, S. J. Perspectives on postdoctoral training: the need for interdisciplinary multidimensional training in mental health. *Menninger Clinic Monographs*, 1973, **17**, 44–57.
10. Grinker, R. R., Sr. Biomedical education as a system. *Arch. Gen. Psychiatry*, 1971, **24**, 291–297.

11. Freedman, A. M. Critical psychiatry: a new and necessary school. *Hospital and Community Psychiatry* 1973, **24,** 819–824.
12. Heilbrunner, R. L. The human prospect. *The New York Review of Books,* 1974, **20,** 21–35.
13. Russell, B. *The impact of science on society.* New York: Columbia University Press, 1951.

NAME INDEX

Adams, J., 147
Albee, G., 221
Alexander, F., 13, 151, 152, 153
Amatruda, C., 206
Anthony, E. J., 87
Apter, N., 179
Arthur, R. J., 235
Ashby, W. R., 115
Astrup, C., 237

Bailey, P., 121
Baldwin, A. L., 172
Basch, M., 123
Bateson, G., 12, 205
Basowitz, H., 166
Beck, S. J., 180
Bender, L., 206
Benedek, T., 64
Benjamin, J. D., 42
Bennett, J. G., 53
Berry, R., 207
Bertalanffy, L. M., 46
Bell, N. W., 134
Bentley, A. F., 73
Beres, D., 128, 169
Betz, B. J., 218
Blatt, S. J., 238
Bleuler, E., 178
Bleuler, M., 178
Boulding, K., 46
Bowlby, J., 120
Branch, J. D., 106
Brodie, H. K. H., 236

Brody, S., 206
Bruner, J., 94
Burnham, D. L., 204

Campbell, M., 183
Cantril, H., 18
Caws, P., 55
Cerralza, M., 238
Child, C. M., 45
Ciba Foundation Conference, 227
Clauson, J. A., 138
Coelho, G. V., 43, 143
Colby, K. M., 125, 127
Coleman, M., 197
Cooper, B., 137
Cottle, T. J. L., 136
Crayton, J., 110

Dewey, J., 73
Diesenhaus, H. I., 76
Dubos, R., 41
Dunham, H. W., 136, 207

Eissler, K. R., 127, 223
Emerson, A., 56
Engel, G., 150
Epstein, S., 197
Erikson, E., 124
Escalona, S., 155, 206

Faris, R. E. L., 136
Feigl, H., 72, 73
Fletcher, J., 218

Frank, J. D., 14
Frankel, C., 17
Frazer, Sir James, 10, 14, 223
Freedman, A., 240
Freedman, D. X., 5, 64, 86, 222, 233
Frenkel-Brunswick, E., 127
Freud, A., 121, 124, 125, 128, 153, 207, 229
Freud, S., 110, 120
Friedenberg, E. Z., 102
Fromm, E., 14

Garber, B., 104
Gedo, J. E., 123, 126
Gesell, A., 206
Giannitrapani, D., 114, 203
Gill, M., 127
Gitelson, M., 121
Globus, G. G., 19
Glover, E., 121
Goldberg, A., 123, 126
Graham, D. T., 152
Grinker, R. R., 28, 29, 102, 121, 135, 139, 152, 163, 167, 168, 199, 241–244
Hamburg, B., 147
Hamburg, D. A., 94, 131, 143, 147
Harlow, H., 120
Harrow, M., 186
Hartman, H., 121
Heath, R., 203
Heider, G. M., 206
Heilbrunner, R. L., 240
Herrick, C. J., 45, 230
Heynes, R., 95
Hilgard, E. R., 163
Hippocrates, 24, 220
Holland, H., 25, 150
Holley, J. W., 209
Hollingshead, A. B., 137
Holzman, P., 126, 127, 163, 197, 199, 203, 204, 207
Hook, S., 125
Hughes, J., 203
Huxley, Sir Julian, 13

Jackson, H., 45
James, William, 119
Janis, I. L., 42
Johnson, C. S., 217
Jones, F. H., 185

Kallman, F., 111, 200
Kaplan, A., 38, 73, 88, 93
Kardiner, A., 127
Kayton, L., 114, 203, 207
Kellam, S. G., 106
Kety, S. S., 111, 113, 200, 202
Kierkegaard, S. A., 221
Klein, G., 26
Kluckhohn, C., 16
Kluckhohn, F., 17
Koch, S., 39
Koestler, A., 43
Koh, S., 207
Kraepelin, E., 34, 35
Kringlen, E., 200

Lazarus, A., 146
Lazlo, E., 45
Levin, F., 147
Levy, L., 136, 137, 139
Lidz, T., 205
Lippitt, R., 95

Maini, S. M., 65
Mandell, A. J., 114
Margenau, H., 28
Maslow, A. G., 35, 228, 229
Masserman, J. H., 69
Mayman, M., 124, 126
Meehl, P., 127, 177
Meltzer, H., 110
Menninger, K., 73
Metzger, W., 33
Millet, J., 121
Millikan, R. A., 15
Millon, T., 44, 76, 124
Minuchin, A., 136, 151
Mishler, E. G., 205
Moos, R., 146
Morgan, H. C., 137
Murphy, G., 43

Murphy, L., 147
Murray, H., 16

Nilsson, J. K., 209
Nordbeck, B., 65
Nurnberger, J. I., 172

Offer, D., 5, 64, 86, 103, 167, 172, 233

Parsons, T., 56, 133
Pearson, K., 18
Peterfreund, E., 126
Piaget, J., 120, 164, 172
Procter, H., 203
Pumpian-Mindlin, E., 127

Rainer, J. D., 109, 110
Ramot, J., 220
Rapaport, D., 45, 126
Redlich, F. C., 137
Rimaldi, H. S., 164
Roback, A. A., 25
Rodnick, E. H., 163
Rogers, C., 15, 35
Romano, J., 238
Rosenthal, A., 5, 200
Roth, J. A., 102
Rowitz, L., 136, 137
Rubinstein, E. A., 43
Reusch, J., 43, 126, 152

Sabshin, M., 103, 220, 236
Sargent, H. D., 89, 123
Schafer, R., 126
Schildkraut, J. J., 111, 202
Selye, H., 143–144
Serota, H. M., 203
Shakow, D., 65, 119, 120, 126, 204, 206
Shands, Harley, 13, 16
Shepherd, M., 53
Sher, J., 44

Sherrington, C., 128
Silber, E., 102
Simpson, G. G., 15, 41
Skinner, B. F., 42
Smelzer, N., 39
Spiegel, J., 47, 134
Spitz, R. A., 120, 152
Spohn, H. E., 204
Stanford University, 143
Strauss, A., 219
Strupp, H. H., 35, 71, 218
Sullivan, H. S., 97, 127
Szent-Gyorgyi, A., 226

Tagiuri, R., 94
Thompson, L., 135
Timberlake, J., 167

Vale, J. R., 115
Vigotsky, L. S., 164

Wallerstein, R., 39
Waxler, N. E., 205
Werble, B., 104, 168
Weiss, P., 38, 46
Whitehead, A. N., 18
Whitehorn, J. C., 218
W.H.O. See World Health Organization
Whorf, B. L., 164
Whyte, L. L., 150
Williams, R. J., 115
Wilson, C., 226
Winokur, G., 112, 113
Wolf, G. H., 151
Wolpert, E. A., 111
World Health Organization, 44
Wynne, L. C., 205

Yi-Chiang, L., 208

Zubin, J., 40

SUBJECT INDEX

Adaptation
 biological mechanisms, 144
 principle of, 121
 study of, 148
 use of term, 143
Adolescent, life style and
 differentiation of organism,
 84
Adolescent rebellion, and
 interest in science, 62–63
Adult, young, as fourth phase
 of life cycle, 84
Age of onset, of schizophrenia,
 190–191
Aging, as fifth phase of life
 cycle, 84
American Psychiatric
 Association, nosological
 classification of, 137
Analogies, as approaches to
 problems, 52, 56
Analogue computer, as creation
 of symbolic thought, 52
Anhedonia. See Pleasureless
 demeanor
Animal drives, vs. humanism,
 154
Antipsychiatry, and
 schizophrenia as
 nondisease, 200
Antiscientism, 12, 227, 233
Anthropology, as part of
 psychiatric system, 224

Anxiety
 neurotic vs. schizophrenic,
 195
 as a system, 178, 193
 in schizophrenia, 187, 189,
 191, 193, 195–196, 197,
 198
Applied science, psychiatry
 viewed as, 70
Aretueus of Cappadox,
 classification of mental
 disorders, 24
Asylum-hospitals, 19th century,
 34
Autism, childhood, vs.
 schizophrenia, 205
Autoimmune disorder, and
 schizophrenia, 202
Autonomy, of investigator, 86

Behavior(s)
 aggressive, two categories of,
 133
 analysis of, 42
 as basic data of psychiatry,
 170
 deviant, interest of scholars
 in, 33
 as focus of psychiatric
 research, 76
 as field for future study,
 122–123

language of use in all
    disciplines, 39
learned, 115
meaning of term, 77
observation of, as keystone of
    psychiatric research, 72
verbal and gross, in study of
    schizophrenia, 210
of young schizophrenics, 191
Behavioral science
    clinical research as, 161
    ideational elements in, 93
    need for research in, 65
    proliferation of theories in,
        73
    psychiatry as part of, 54, 223
Behavioral therapy, regarded as
    short-cut, 226
Behaviorism, 41
"Behavior-observation-
    inference" model, 90
Bias, in psychoanalytic studies,
    120
Biochemical substances, in
    development of psychoses,
    113
Biochemist, and clinical
    phenomena, 40
Biofeedback techniques, 42
Biological factors, in mental
    disturbances, 110
Biology
    and the humanities, 41
    and schizophrenia, 192,
        200–204
Biometric model, 40
Blacks, and mental illness, 137
Borderline syndrome, 19, 42,
    104
Boundaries, semipermeable, of
    living systems, 50
Brain damage
    and schizophrenia, 115
    predisposition to, 202
    and twin studies, 111
Bridging work
    in psychiatric research, 87

and schizophrenia, 210
in stress research, 147
Bureaucrats
    in psychiatry, 226
    regulating research, 238

Catecholamines, in twin
    studies, 111
Central nervous system
    in schizophrenia, 205
    catecholamine metabolism,
        202
Cerebral cortex, regulatory
    function of, 49
Chicago area research, 136
Child development studies
    observations in, 120
    and study of neuroses, 155
    use of video tape, 119
Childhood, as second phase of
    life cycle, 83
Childhood schizophrenics, 206
Child psychiatrists, attitudes to
    research, 87
Children, "high-risk," 206
Chimpanzees,
    destructive-aggression in,
    132–133
Classifications (of mental
    disorders), 24
    American and International
        systems, 75
    beginnings of, 73
    behavioral analysis as
        alternative to, 42
    confused, and need for
        research, 75
    difficulty of, 55
    as first step toward scientific
        psychiatry, 177
    inaccuracy of, 44
    inadequacy of, 176
    as major preoccupation, 34
    needed to develop
        hypotheses, 81
    of schizophrenia, 178–183

Clinical investigations, general systems theory in, 56
Clinical psychiatrists, and interest in research, 74–75
Clinical psychiatry, 6
  vs. research psychiatry, 223
  as science, 36
  vs. psychiatry as science, 55
Clinical psychologist, sketch of, 26–27
Clinical research
  on schizophrenia, 180
  work-outline, 181–182
Clinical syndrome, problem of definition, 171
Clinicians
  and empirical and statistical findings, 96
  as obstructionists to research, 87
Coherence, organizational, and schizophrenia, 188
Communication(s)
  considered core of psychiatry, 71
  lack of, and anxiety, 195–196
  needs of infant, 61–62
  personal, Kohut's definition of, 17
  systems, defined, 135
  theories of, and energy exchange, 50
Communicative behavior, and thought disorder, 188
Community mental health centers, 106
Community psychiatry, 37, 106, 234
Competence, deficiency in, in schizophrenia, 190
Computer analysis, of research data, 92
Conflict, as essence of life, 144
Control function, of human being, 175–176

Control
  of higher levels over lower levels, 50
  psychological concept of, 50
Controls
  in clinical research, 167
  normal, 101
Coping behavior, 146, 147, 148, 149
Coping devices
  learning of, 84
  social standards for, 219
Coping, use of term, 143
Cortical response, in schizophrenics, 203
Crash programs, public demand for, 234
Creativity, innate, families and, 62
Cross-sectional approach, vs. longitudinal, 167
Culture
  change under stress, 135
  as human specialization, 133
Curability, cult of, 25
Custodial care, beginnings of, 25

Data
  amount of, in research, 89
  analyst of, inclusion in research plan, 92
  collection method, 93, 94
  retrospective, inaccuracy of, 93
Death, as later phase in life cycle, 84
de Chardin, Teilhard, quoted on science and faith, 15
Dedifferentiation, biological, 9
Defense, use of term, 143
Defenses, in schizophrenia, 193, 195
Defensive lifestyle, 154
Dementia praecox
  classification of Kraepelin,

75, 178
use of term, 38
Demography
  and mental disorders, 136
  studies of schizophrenia, 208
Demonic possession, and
  psychotic behavior, 34
Dependency, excessive, in
  schizophrenia, 189
Depression
  age of onset, 112
  biological factors in, 112, 113
  in creative scientists, 63
  initiation of process, 40
Descartes, René, and dichotomy
  of external and inner
  reality, 26
Devolution, Jacksonian, 9
Diagnosis
  deficient interest in, 222
  importance of, 177
  and psychiatric research, 74
Diathesis-stress model, 201
Differentiation process and
  parts of system, 48, 49
Digital spectrum analysis, in
  schizophrenia, 114
"Dilution," writings on,
  124–125
Dimethyltryptamine, in
  schizophrenia, 202
Disease, in life style of aging,
  84
Distress, personal, as indication
  for psychotherapy, 70–71
Dopamine, overactivity of, and
  schizophrenia, 202
Dostoevski, expression of
  revolt, 13
"Drift" hypothesis, 136–137
  and schizophrenia, 207–208
Drive quantities, in chronic
  schizophrenia, 197
Drive theories, psychologists
  and, 164
Drugs, psychotropic, 114, 220

discovery of, 110
early bias against, 220
misuse of, 234
use of, in 19th century, 25,
  34
Dual instinct theory, 121

Ecology
  of community, and frequency
    of mental disorder, 137
  social, of mental illness,
    138
Economic status, and choice of
  goals, 62
Education
  early, and creative potential,
    67
  social, and prevention of
    mental illness, 139
  therapeutic activity system as,
    70
Ego depletion syndrome, 49
Ego functions
  and behavior analysis, 42
  Beres enumeration, 169–170
  expressed as behaviors,
    170–171
Ego psychology, era of, 121
Electrodes, use in studying
  schizophrenics, 203
Electroencephelogram
  and schizophrenia, 202–203
  and other diseases, 114
Electroshock therapy, 220
Ellipsis, 187
Emotion-judging task and
  reliability of observation,
    94
Empathy, through expansion of
  self, 17
Empirical approach, to unity of
  science, 55
Empirical phenomena, as test
  of knowledge, 51
Empirical research, relation to
  theory, 38
"Encounter" groups, 221

Enlightenment, 18th century, and treatment of psychotics, 25
Entities, psychiatric, shifting nature of, 234–235
Environment(s)
  changing, and coping devices, 194
  as factor in development, 83
  and schizophrenia, 201
  as source of stress-stimuli, 134
Epidemiology, and mental disease, 136, 138, 139, 235
Epinephrine, producing anxiety, 197
Epistemology, current problems of, 28
Ethical problems, for psychiatry, 227
Ethics, and human behavior, 16–17
Etiological approach to neuroses, 153
Etiologies of schizophrenia, 182
Evolution, and religion, 15
Exogenous conditions, separated from endogenous, 36
Exorcism, 23–24
Experiences, environmental and differentiation of organism, 83
Experimental method, in investigations, 166–167
Existentialist psychiatrist, 221
Eye movements, of schizophrenics, 203

Facts, relation to ideas, 29–30
Faith vs. science, 12
  and mental health, 230
Family(ies)
  and child's scientific attitude, 62
  in clinical research, 171
  as communications system,

and genesis of schizophrenia, 204, 205
  disturbed, 134
  shift from extended to nuclear, 235
  of schizophrenics, 201
Family life, and schizophrenia, 179
Family therapy, 221
Fantasy life, and interest in research, 63
Federal law, specifications on research projects, 91–92
Feedback deficit, Holzman's theory of, 197
Feeling, and nature of reality, 14·
Follow-up, in long-term research, 104, 167
"Four A's" of schizophrenia (Bleuler's), 178
Fragmentation, feeling of, in schizophrenia, 191
Freud, Anna, 128
Freud, Sigmund
  concept of neuroses, 154
  deifying of, 223
  dual instinct theory, 125
  principle of conflict, 153
  and psychodynamic psychology, 229
  and schizophrenias, 207
  theoretical development of, 121
  theory of unconscious mental processes, 124
Freudian ideas, and current analytic theory, 37
Funds, for psychiatric research, 233, 238
Futurology, 109, 233

Gandhi, Mahatma, psychological control of, 50
GAP reports, 64, 65, 76

Genealogical studies, in
   schizophrenia, 200
General Adaptation Syndrome,
   of Selye, 144
General systems theory, 46, 47
   criticisms of, 52–53
   and psychoanalysts, 127
   and psychoanalytic theory, 56
   and schizophrenia, 208
Genetics
   behavioral, 131
   and environment,
      interlocking of, 110
   influence on development,
      82, 83
   and manic-depressives, 112
   and premorbid personality,
      182
   and psychiatry, 109
   and schizophrenia, 200
Gestalt, spectrum of theories
   as, 47
Goals
   of psychiatric research, 78
   sought by man, 51
   of therapies, 70
Gods, as successors to magic,
   11
Governmental funding and
   interest in research, 88–89
Governmental support,
   declining, 233, 236
Grants, training, for psychiatric
   residents, 74
Greek philosophers, concerns
   of, 23
Grinker, R. R., career of,
   241–244
Group membership roles, 134
Group therapy, 221

Health
   defined, 218
   factors in, 104
Health-illness system,
   development and decline
   in, 104

Heterogeneous syndrome,
   schizophrenia as, 192
Hierarchies, dependence on
   control, 50
Homeostatic functions, 49
Homeostatic regulation,
   deficient, in schizophrenia,
   204
Homoclites, use of term, 102,
   149
Hospitalization, in
   schizophrenia, 190
Hospital records, as research
   data, 92–93
Human subject, and psychiatric
   research, 92, 161
Human system, analysis of, 85
Humanism
   new, 223
   and psychiatric science, 20
   vs. science, 12
Hydrocorticosteroids (17) in
   depression, 112, 113
Hypnosis, in clinical research,
   163
Hypothalamus, and abnormal
   biochemical activity, 202
Hypotheses
   defined, 38
   testing of, 78–79
   psychoanalytic, 125
Hypothetical constructs, in
   psychiatric research, 81

Identity crisis, of psychiatric
   profession, 236
Illness, defined, 218
Individuality, increasing, of
   man, 82
Infant(s)
   in first phase of life cycle, 83
   oral needs of, and drive for
      knowing, 61
   and prediction of neurotic
      disturbances, 206
   "soft" neurological signs in,
      202

Inference, degree of, and reliability of observation, 95

Information, in open systems, 50

Informed consent, 92, 167, 183, 238

Initiation rites, as magical thinking, 10

Instinctual processes, and health vs. pathology, 122

Instrument, law of, by Kaplan, 88

Integration, of psychiatric system, 176–177

Integrity, systems for maintaining, 175

Intelligence, of schizophrenics, 190

Interviews
in clinical research, 162
schizophrenia research, 182
"depth," vs. behavioral data, 72

Introspection
in ancient philosophies, 24
in psychoanalysis, 124

Introvert, vs. extrovert, as potential research worker, 63

Investigator
formulation of conclusions, 96–97
motivation of, 88
need for clinical training, 66
need for cooperation, 86, 87
personality of, 65
professional qualifications of, 64–65
selection and development of, 67–68

I.Q. test, 162

Irrationalism, as studied attitude '17–18

Isolation, as stimulus for anxiety, 195–196

Isomorphism, of living systems, 52, 55

Jefferson, Thomas, psychological control of, 50

Knowledge, pathways to, 15

Koch, postulates for bacterial disease, 178

Kraepelin, classification of, 24, 34–35, 3, 110, 178

L-dopa, and depression, 113

Learning
extrinsic vs. personal, 228
laws of, and behavior analysis, 41
ontological phases of, 28

Learning theory, absent in psychoanalysis, 126

Libido, in psychoanalytic theory, 122

Life cycle, phases in, 104, 105
as area of research, 172
and coping, 145–146
in developing theory, 175
and diagnosis and treatment, 36
interdependence of, 239

Life style
and health, 149
phases of, 83–84
semicircular diagram of, 84–85

Literature search, importance in research, 78, 90

Luther, Martin, psychological control of, 50

Magic
as manipulation of nature, 10
related to science, 9
in religion and psychiatry, 223

Maimonides, on creative research, 67

Man
  contradictory movement
    through life, 16
  higher nature of, 229
Manic-depression
  vs. depression, 112
  and norepinephrine, 111
"Mankind" concept, 218
Mathematics, replacing
  philosophy, 26
Mathematization, premature, of
  general systems theory, 53
Maturation process, and
  environment, 43
Maturity, and unfinished world
  view, 73
Medical education, shortening
  of, 238
Medical model
  acceptance by psychologists,
    26
  based on classification, 75
  vs. humanistic model, 35
  vs. socioeducational model,
    65
  strict adherants of, 220
Mental disorders
  ancient approach to, 23–24
  classifications of, 24
Mental health, determined by
  society, 219
Mental illness, prevention of,
  237
Metatheory, general systems
  theory as, 47
Methods, in psychiatric
  research, 81
Milieu, social and cultural, and
  health and illness, 131
Milieu therapy, 221
  as new form of moral
    therapy, 37
Mind, evolution of, 12
"Mind-body" problem, 149,
  150
"Mission-oriented" research,
  78, 88–89, 234

Mitchell, Weir, rest cures of,
  25, 34
MMPI, 162
Model building, theoretical, 46
Models, of mind, and
  psychoanalytic theories,
  123
Money, as motive for research,
  88
Monotheism, beginnings of, 11
"Moral" (humane) treatment of
  mental patients, 34, 35
Mother-infant relationship, 131
Multidisciplinary conference,
  on coping and adaptation,
  143
Multidisciplinary group, and
  schizophrenia, 206
Multidisciplinary research, 37,
  39, 44, 54, 77, 91, 165,
  238–241
  and psychoanalysis, 126
Multidisciplinary viewpoint, 135
Mystical concepts, and clinical
  research, 171
Mysticism
  and science, 19
  two forms of, 223

"Naming is knowing," 73
National Institute for Mental
  Health Research Study
  Group, 74
  and researchers in psychiatry,
  67
Naturalists, influence on
  process concepts, 45
Nature vs. nurture dichotomy,
  43, 110
Negentrophy, 64
Neologisms, 187
Neophobia, 206
Nervous system, evolution of,
  45
  Jacksonian concept, 50
Neuropathology, modern, 110
  as "queen of sciences," 25

Neuroses
  biogenic basis for, 155
  research on, 153
Neurotics, 19th century
  threatment of, 34
Nissl and Alzheimer, work of,
  109
Norepinephrine, effect on
  emotions, 111
Normal, neglect of, 149
Normality, 101–107, 149
  four perspectives on, 103
  social standards of, 219
  W. H. O. definition of, 44
Nosology. See Classifications

Objectivity
  inseparable from subjectivity,
    230
  in scientific investigator, 66
Observations, in
    psychoanalysis, 125
  and reliability, definition of
    unit, 95
    importance of training, 96
  in psychiatric research,
    94–95
Observers, types of, 166
Obsessive-compulsive
    personalities, as magical
    thinking, 10
Occupational rituals, as magical
    thinking, 10
Ontogeny, as subsystem in life
    cycle, 105, 175
Ontology
  of phases of learning, 28
  philosophy of, and study of
    life cycle, 85
Organic syndromes, separation
    from functional, 35
Organic systems, effect of
    stress-responses, 144
Organism, living
  as open system, 134
  transactions of somatic and
    psychic systems, 49

Outcome theory, 37–38
Overexcitement, autonomic, in
    schizophrenics, 204
Overinclusion, conceptual,
    186–187

Parents
  of schizophrenics, 201
    interference from, 205
Parochialism of psychoanalysis,
    37
Pathways, final common, of
    Jackson, 45
Patience, needed in research,
    64
Peptic ulcer, Mirsky's model,
    151
Personality
  and constitution, 115
  interaction with social
    systems, 135
  premorbid, of schizophrenia,
    182
  study of, 163
Personality characteristics
    reciprocal relationship, 224
Personality deviations, and
    psychiatric research, 42
Phasic evolutions, of
    schizophrenics, 179
Phenothiazines, first
    appearance of, 220
Philosophy
  and evolution of scientific
    thinking, 33
  relation to psychology, 24
Physician-philosopher, first
    appearance of, 24
Physiology, effect on mind, 237
Pilot study, as step in research
    design, 92–93
Plan, importance in research
    design, 91
Plasma protein factor, in
    schizophrenia, 202
Play, research work as, 63

Pleasure, equated with coping behavior, 147
Pleasureless demeanor, of schizophrenia, 189
Pluralism, 43, 225
Polygenetic theory, vs. Mendelian inheritance, 201
Poverty, and schizophrenia, 137
Pragmatic approach, 26
Prediction, in personality-theoretical research, 42–43
Prestige, as incentive for research, 63
Primates, study of, 133
Privacy, invasion of, in direct observation methods, 119–120
Problem-solving, mathematical vs. systematic approach, 53
Process, vs. content, in clinical research programs, 57
Prospective methods, for studying schizophrenia, 185
Protean manifestations of schizophrenia, 184
Psychiatrists
needed in research, 76
opinions on social issues, 226
and science-humanism conflict, 20
two groups of, 54
Psychiatry
clinical. See Clinical psychiatry
defined, 53, 69
development from philosophy and psychology, 23–31
four areas of data, 81
fragmentation into schools, 35
including all of life, 238
object of inquiry in, 69–79
relation to psychology and philosophy, 165

as science, 36, 53, 222
social. See Social psychiatry
as social science, 217
transcultural, defined, 136
Psychic energy, 122
vs. physical energy, 128
Psychic evolution, four phases of, 15
Psychoanalysis
effect on nosology, 177
need for scientific methods, 125
and schizophrenia, 207
and sociology, 39
value of, 37
Psychoanalysts
attitude toward theory, 125
hostility to scientific studies, 121
Psychodynamicists, and humanists, 227
Psychological components of schizophrenia, 204–208
Psychologists
clinical, as observers, 161
clinical orientation, 26
in hospitals, 34
role on research team, 165
separation into schools, 24
Psychology
split from philosophy, 33
state of crisis in, 33–34
Psychopharmacology, 114
and schizophrenia, 202
Psychoses
differentiation of, 179
"irreversible," of Apter, 179
Psychosis, as outcome in schizophrenia, 192
Psychosomatic concepts, early prediction of, 25–26
Psychosomatic illness
and biofeedback techniques, 42
explanatory concepts, 152
Psychosomatic medicine, 37

Psychosomatic, use of term,
150–151
Psychotherapy
as ancient art, 220
relation to magic and
religion, 14
Psychotics, concepts about,
separated from neurotics,
34
Public
and psychiatric research, 234
view of psychiatrists, 219

Questionnaires, in clinical
research, 162, 163

Rating scales, for
schizophrenia, 183
Reaction time, in
schizophrenia, 206
Reality-testing, 169
"Real Self," doctrine of, 228
Reason
as psychological process, 18
revolt against, 10
Reductionism
vs. humanism, 176
in psychiatry, 36, 122
in psychology, 26, 38
Regression
Freudian, 9
psychological and physical,
85
Religion
in ancient thought processes,
23
modern meaning of, 11–12
as psychosocial imperative,
13
related to science, 9
Research
biological, 109–115
clinical, 161–174, 180,
181–182
psychiatric, design of, 81–99
deductive and inductive, 77
four levels of, 136

ideographic and
nomothetic, 77, 82
lack of organization in, 74
limitations of, 166
practical difficulties in, 86
reasons for interest in, 76
psychoanalytic, 124
difficulties of, 127
psychological, and
schizophrenia, 204
Research experiences, early
scientific orientation, 65
Research program, checklist of
questions on, 97–99
Research workers, as group of
psychiatry, 54
Researcher, qualities of, 61–68
Retrospective information,
inaccuracy of, 119
Retrospective methods, for
studying schizophrenia,
185
Revolution, and socio-cultural
environment, 83
Role-identity confusion, in
schizophrenia, 208
Rorschach test, 162, 179
data in schizophrenia
research, 181
Russell, Bertrand, quoted on
future, 244

Schizophrenia, 175–215
classifications of, 178–183
development of, methods of
studying, 185–186
diagnosis of, 179
diagnostic categories,
180–181
manifestations of, 183–192
Michael Reese definition, 210
nonpsychotic forms of, 184,
186
as polygenetic inadequacy,
113
research work-outline,
181–182
subsystems in, 192

Schizoaffective, 179, 181
Schizophrenic patients,
    distinguishing qualities of,
    191
Schizophrenic State Inventory,
    183
Schizophrenic syndrome,
    described, 199
"Schizophrenic spectrum," 201
Schizophrenics, hidden, 201
Schizotaxic individual,
    precipitation into
    psychosis, 199
Schools of thought
    development of, 24, 33, 35,
    37
    in psychology, 164
    and varying diagnoses, 75
Science
    vs. humanism, 227, 229
    and religion, 12
    repudiation of, 9–10. See also
    Antiscientism
Science of Systematics, 73
Scientific attitude, in children,
Scientific career, qualities
    needed, 66
Scientific discipline, psychiatry
    as, 35
Scientific method, 18
Scientific progress, enemies of,
    18
Scientific truths, and common
    sense, 73
Scientist, and abstract
    conceptualization, 28
Self-esteem, challenge to, and
    schizophrenia, 190
Serendipity, importance in
    research, 64
Set theory of schizophrenia, of
    Shakow, 206
Shakow, D., clinical research of,
    166
Shifting, of schizophrenic
    symptomatology, universal
    and individual, 198–199

Siblings, of schizophrenics, 201
Signal anxiety, 194, 196
Six Schizophrenias (Beck), 180
"Skidrow" areas,
    schizophrenics in, 207–208
Sleep rhythm, disturbed, in
    schizophrenia, 202
"Slippage" of thought, in
    schizophrenia, 187
Social change, rapid, and
    disturbed families, 134
Social class, and frequency of
    mental disorder, 137
    lower, and schizophrenia,
    208
Social life, and individual
    gratification, 105
Social psychiatry, 236
    defined, 136
    relevance of, 106
Social techniques, and
    psychiatry, 131–139
Social turbulence and stress
    responses, 139
Social workers, in clinical
    research, 163
Society
    held responsible for man's
    problems, 44
    low regard for abstractions,
    225–226
    and personality development,
    105
    role of psychiatry in,
    217–232
Socio-cultural studies, of
    schizophrenia, 207
Socioeconomic status, lower,
    treatment of patients, 221
Sociology, as part of psychiatric
    system, 224
Sociotherapists, 221
Somatotherapists, 220
Sources, primary, importance
    to investigator, 90
Specificity, response theory of,
    106

SSI. *See* Schizophrenic State
    Inventory
Straight evolutions, of
    schizophrenia, 178–179
Stress, 143–157
  and thought disorders, 188
Stress experiments, normal
    controls in, 102
Stress research, 37
Stress-responses, 145
  and research, 78
Stress stimuli, causing
    dedifferentiation, 48
"Stress tolerance test," 163
Statistician, and data analysis,
    96
  on research team, 168
Suicide, as shortcut in life
    cycle, 85
"Sulk-prone" child, and
    development of
    depression, 114
Symbolic system, Grinker's
    phases of, 28
Symbolic systems, man's
    creation of, 51
Symbols, role in science, 27
Symptomatology, of
    schizophrenia, 177–192
System, collapse of, 176
  problem of systematic study
    of, 41
Systems approach
  to psychiatry, 175
  to schizophrenia, 200, 204

Tape recording
  of clinical interview,
    182–183, 187
  in psychoanalytic
    observation, 125, 127
"Target" research. *See*
    "Mission-oriented"
    research
Taxonomy, problems of, 235
Teachers, influence on future
    research workers, 63

Teleology, function of, 51
Terry lectures
  of 1927, 15
  of 1949, 15
Tests
  in clinical research, 162
    reliability of, 168
  in schizophrenia, 179, 209
Theory(ies)
  based on observed facts, 28
  defined, 38
  differentiated from model, 43
  general, development of, 82
  integrated, development of,
    175–215
  in psychoanalytic literature,
    123
  and testable hypotheses, 52
  tested against facts, 73
Therapist(s)
  vs. investigator, differential
    features of, 64
  as group of psychiatrists, 54
Therapy, kinds of, 35
Thinking
  idiosyncratic, in
    schizophrenia, 186
  personalized, 186
  unitary, 29, 46, 240
Third Force psychology, 229
Thought, Frazer's web of, 14
Thought disorder, in
    schizophrenia, 179, 186
Thought processes, ancient,
    three phases of, 23
Thoughts, intertwined with
    feelings, 15
Thyroid deficiency, and
    catatonia, 202
Transactionalism, 71
Transactional research, 82
Transactions, observations of,
    19
Transcendental reality, 13–14
Transmethylization, disturbance
    in, 202
Traumatic anxiety, 194

Treatment, as separate function
from research, 171
Tripartite structural theory, 121
Twin studies
monozygotic and dizygotic,
111
and schizophrenia, 200

Uncertainty principle, of
Heisenberg, 3
Unified approach, to
schizophrenia research,
208–211
Unifying theories, development
of, 46
Unity of science, 55
Utopia, expectations of, 14

Value, judgments of, 188,
19
Value-orientations, 16–17
five questions, on, 17

Value systems
regressions in, 10
of science, 12
Video-tape recording, in
observation of child
development, 119
Vitamin deficiency, and
schizophrenia, 202
Vocabularies
as barriers to communication,
39, 44
and multidisciplinary
research, 91
in psychiatry, 218

Web-of-life concept, 135, 136
Wisdom, conventional,
challenged by investigator,
64
Witchcraft, identified with
psychotic behavior, 34
World War II, postwar
advances in research, 74